Reinventing Retirement: How To Make Your Golden Years Fulfilling, Rewarding And Fun

Reinventing Retirement
How To Make Your Golden Years Fulfilling, Rewarding And Fun

V. P. Sarin

MEGAGEM

Published by MegageM Sapience
www.megagem.org
gem@megagem.org
ISBN-13: 9788192777214
ISBN-10: 8192777219

CONTENTS

Preface

Not so long ago, there was no such thing as retirement. Most people worked as long as they were able to work productively. Retirement is a relatively new concept born in Germany in the 1880s and became popular in America during the Great Depression of the 1930s. Before the advent of the concept of retirement, old people were not sidelined. Rather, they were greatly valued for their knowledge and experience. They were respected as a resource for their insight, wisdom and common sense.

After remaining fairly constant for most of human history, average human longevity has nearly doubled since the beginning of the idea of retirement. Another thing that remained constant for most of human history was that our population always formed a sort of pyramid with young children making the base and each older cohort serially representing a smaller and smaller unit on top of that. But the population patterns, particularly in developed countries, no longer form a pyramid. There are as many older people as the younger ones. But then, we often pay no heed to these two relevant factors while discussing retirement planning or the golden years of our life.

We need to redefine and reinvent our own concept of retirement to befit our vision of the golden years. Some senior people are retiring old notions of what it means to be retired. They are reinventing retirement to recharge and revitalise their lives. They are pursuing their productive passions that draw on the skills, talents and wisdom they have acquired all through their lives. They are listening to the call of their cherished calling to rediscover retirement. They want to treat, not retreat. They want to rewire, not retire.

But then, many people are not amenable to the new situation. They are not ready to confidently stand up to the pulls and pressures of a phlegmatic society. They don't realise that retirement is actually the time to put in practice all the lessons learned in their lives. They don't appreciate that having a constructive mission can make a big difference in their lives.

Your life has no meaning if you are not happy and cannot make others happy. It is not an either/or choice. The right retirement strategy aims at a synergistic approach to seek the both. It expects us to clear the decks at the conceptual level. Otherwise, our unbridled quest for success would only drag us deeper into the retirement dilemmas.

You should treat your retirement decisions just as seriously as any other part of your life. And it is important to be in control of your retirement decisions. This book lets you take responsibility for your future. It aims to create a success-consciousness within you, which empowers you to control your future rather than letting your future control you. It provides enough inputs to enable you to effectively deal with your retirement dilemmas so that you can smartly monitor your future to ensure your wholesome happiness. It helps you explore some pragmatic strategies to exploit your latent talents, which in turn, will help you release the negative, stay positive and enrich your life in the process. You just have to join the dots to figure out the holistic way to health, wealth and happiness.

I dedicate this book to my daughter Priya Sarin, who is yet to start her career but still wanted to redact and edit this retirement manual. I asked her to keep this book simple, practical and just relevant to real retirement issues. We also consciously decided to reiterate a few known points to draw on the power of your sub-conscious with the intention of realising the context-relevant objectives. And to provide purpose, direction and motivation to the readers, Priya added some examples of contemporary illustrious leaders after taking their permission. Instead of hanging their boots or slowing down after formal retirement, these eminent exemplars like Dr. Manmohan Singh, Mr. Narayana Murthy and Mr. Ratan Tata began their next innings with renewed zest and zeal. Even after winding down their careers, they still prefer to stay in the game for the benefit of the society.

The central theme of this book is to encourage people to draw on their abilities to make the most of their professional and personal lives during retirement. The objective is to encourage readers to avail the benefits of working after formal retirement. The credit for many features aimed at improving the psychological impact of the material, at times even at the expense of syntax, goes to my friends who have tested this material and offered their valuable feedback and comments to make this work more practical and useful. The objective is to ensure that it empowers you to manage your future successfully and you are amply motivated to take your retirement decisions realistically and intelligently. Constructive suggestions to further improve the book are most welcome.

I hope it will help you to reflect on your retirement issues and opportunities. I pray that God allows you to change for the better to have a blessed retirement life so that it will be the best part of your life.

Let's get ready for a great retirement. Let's reinvent your golden years.

V. P. Sarin

Retirement Myths And Realities

Retirement, as we understand it today, is not a natural part of our life cycle. The idea of retirement didn't really exist in the pre-industrial era. It is the unique creation of the industrial age. Earlier, people used to work till almost the fag end of their lifetime. But then, they rarely lived past today's retirement age.

Today again, many retirees are taking the same path, but not because life ceases before retirement, but because life goes on after retirement. Most of them think life has no meaning, value or purpose without work. Dr. Ken Dychtwald, an ageing expert and best-selling author of sixteen books on ageing-related issues, says that people now see retirement as a time for new priorities, new opportunities and new strategies for today's challenges. Today most people consider retirement as a new beginning, not just a winding down. They prefer to work in retirement 'to stay active and involved.'

Retirement is more a state of mind than a stage of life. Most experts feel that the concept of retirement has outlived its intended purpose. In the modern world, they feel the concept of retirement is no longer relevant in its current format.

Today we ought to question the very assumptions on which the idea of retirement was built. It seems the only thing that needs retiring is the current concept of retirement itself. In fact, retirement is a myth in today's tech-driven world. Before we try to demystify this myth, let's first analyse some most common retirement myths so as to bring reality into focus.

👤 👤 👤 Myth: People should stop working once they retire.

☑☑☑ Reality: We should enjoy our work as long as we want. We ought to rewire, not retire. It is not merely because we are living longer and need to finance our additional years. It is primarily because we typically have a natural need to contribute something as long as we live. This need to add value to our life as well as to those around us does not cease at a preset age, that too usually determined by others.

Retirement is not a destination; it's a journey. Life

continues after retirement. And sticking to a routine has great benefits. The objective of retirement planning is not just to provide income needed to support your desired retirement lifestyle. Working after you achieve your financial freedom has many non-monetary benefits. Your cognitive ageing slows down when you are gainfully employed. Research says that if you work longer, you can experience a happier, healthier and more fulfilling life in retirement. Remember that purpose and meaning in life is what keeps us going.

🗣🗣🗣 Myth: Retirement is exclusively a financial event. Money is everything when it comes to retirement planning.

❓☑❓☑ Reality: When it comes to retirement, planning is everything. And money is only a part of the bigger picture. In fact, the lifestyle decisions are one of the most important concerns for your retirement years. And money is just one of the means to find meaning in your later years. So you need to focus as carefully on your retirement lifestyle planning as you focus on money.

🗣🗣🗣 Myth: For most people, retirement is just associated with poor physical and mental health after retirement.

❓☑❓☑ Reality: Just retirement does not lead to a decline in health or life satisfaction for most people.

For years, scientists have been trying to understand whether retirement is good for health, bad for it, or neutral. For many people, retirement is associated with improvement in health. But others feel that retirement is a frustrating period marked by declining health. Generally, people who know how to make good use of their time experience positive changes.

While it may be interesting to understand how retirement affects people, it has nothing to do with how it will affect you. After all, it is in your control to make the retirement years the best years of your life.

👤 👤 👤 Myth: My health insurance will pay all my medical bills.

❓☑❓☑ Reality: People often think that health insurance will cover most health care expenses. But health insurance doesn't cover everything. Without proper planning, uncovered health care and allied costs could be a major part of the annual budget in retirement.

👤 👤 👤 Myth: My retirement won't last that long

❓☑❓☑ Reality: Life expectancy is rising fast. And this trend is expected to continue in the coming years. But then, this good news also signals a need for extra retirement income. Thanks to advances in medicine and healthier lifestyles, you may live longer than you think.

👤👤👤 Myth: I can depend on my family and/or government for support in retirement.

❓☑❓☑ Reality: One cannot depend on anyone else for support in retirement. Some people use this as an excuse to delay their retirement planning. In fact, no one wants to become a dependant on other family members in their retirement years. As a matter of fact, people want true financial independence in their sunset years. It is important to understand that if you want to enjoy retirement years, you will have to plan and arrange funds and other resources yourself.

👤👤👤 Myth: My living expenses after retirement will be lower.

❓☑❓☑ Reality: Many people believe that their living expenses will be lower in retirement and will continue to decrease over time. The general rule of thumb that you will need roughly 70% of your pre-retirement income to maintain a similar lifestyle may not be true. This assumption does not take into account more free time and more leisure choices. It may be true if you spend less during holidays. But remember, making wrong assumptions regarding your retirement plan can make it all the more difficult to retire well.

👤👤👤 Myth: Most people work after retirement because they need money.

❶☑❷☑ Reality: A new Merrill Lynch study indicates that most people do not work after retirement for money. This study has again confirmed that most people work after retirement *to stay mentally active*. Surprisingly *money* was at no. 4, after *to stay physically active* and *sense of identity/self worth*. The AARP Working in Retirement Study also showed similar findings.

In fact, the majority of people (80%) work after retirement because they *want to*, rather than because they *have to*.

Many people are not able to view retirement in the right perspective owing to several myths associated with it. They often fall prey to these common myths and give up their positive way of thinking. So, it is always better to first examine and replace these myths with facts so as to create a receptive mood.

And by no means, the above mentioned myths make an exhaustive list of retirement myths. In fact, some other retirement myths may cross your mind when you think about retirement issues. However, you should not get distracted or overwhelmed by them. You can always unravel them if you really want to.

Of course, it's up to you to get the ball rolling. Nobody else is going to do it for you. You have to take personal responsibility for your future. Remember the old saying, "If it's to be, it's up to me."

2

Redefining Retirement

Many middle-aged people, especially the salaried class, take the retirement term literally and unequivocally concede that the professional hibernation is an inescapable destiny. They think that they are predestined to renounce their calling on retirement and can only look forward to their hobbies or other leisure time activities to pass time thereafter. While they mistakenly believe that withdrawal from the active work life is the one and only imminent default option, they also tend to disregard the fact that time utilisation in the post-retirement period is a serious issue with many health, financial, professional and social consequences.

But then, such people ignore that even during retirement, professional and social consequences can be important for them as they are accustomed to a privileged professional status in the society. It is not easy for them to graciously adapt to any change in their professional standing. Retirement planning is an opportunity to focus on health, financial, professional and social challenges ahead and explore the ways to avert them. Today's circumstances call for a holistic approach to retirement planning, not merely to meet the contemporary challenges, but also to make the most of our expertise and lead a happy, purposeful life till the end.

Several studies besides our hands-on experience suggest that even after formal retirement you can opt for a meaningful career to make a big difference in your life as well as those around you. You can contribute a lot to the society with all the knowledge and wisdom acquired by you and while doing so, you can ensure better health and improved quality of life for yourself. Perceived or real concerns relating to later years' work life should not deter you, because when you face your inhibitions about the challenges of the post-retirement professional life and overpower them, you will find that almost all the misperceived hurdles have disappeared. So to get going, you just need to tackle your real issues in a rational and planned way.

You ought to plan for an active work life even if there is no need for financial rewards because many other positive factors, including the eternal human urge to contribute something, call for a positive and practical retirement career planning.

Admittedly, I am somewhat prejudiced towards working during later years but this propensity, perhaps bias, stems from the real life success stories of seniors, who made the most of their later years. To stay active and connected is the secret of these wise people to enjoy the best possible health. They know that a post-retirement career can improve a person's physical, emotional, financial and mental well-being.

Just think about what motivates business leaders like Ratan Tata, Azim Premji and N R Narayan Murthy to actively engage in social causes to make a difference in people's lives. Why they are passionate about their work on issues they feel most strongly about? Because they find spreading happiness around more fulfilling than retirement. That is why they are so passionate about what they do!

When someone asked Amitabh Bachchan on his 71st birthday about his retirement plans, he replied, "I want to work till my last breath." Dr APJ Abdul Kalam, one of India's most loved presidents, kept inspiring people till his last breath. He breathed his last while doing what he loved most – teaching.

You too can find many such exemplars if you look around. I want you to press the accelerator more often than the brakes even in your later years. You may switch to a more reliable vehicle, i.e. work of your choice, but move ahead.

And career planning for later years is equally important, if not more, than the career planning for initial years. Earlier career planning for later years was not so important, because career options for older adults were limited. Also, earlier the needs of the society, as well as individuals, were different. Now experienced people need to realise that the scene is different today, and they owe it to themselves and their loved ones to make the best use of their potential in the larger interests of the society.

The humanity expects and deserves this contribution from seniors especially in the light of rapidly rising proportion of idle seniors' vis-à-vis the working population. Senior people can contribute to this noble cause simply by empowering themselves to continue their career journey as long as they deem fit. This path will also assure a genuine fulfilment and adequate financial security throughout their life. However, we need to prepare ourselves for this exciting journey, because daydreaming or calculations on the back of envelope will not help.

Before we take up the later years career planning, we prefer to consider the following basic factors, which may possibly influence your retirement work plans. These familiar yet frequently forgotten points are purposely configured to stimulate your thought process so as to empower you to plan your future intelligently.

Physical Activity

Moderate physical exercise during later years is not just desired, but is essential to keep ourselves physically fit. As we age, several body parts tend to become less efficient. And physical inactivity accelerates this process. It can even restrict the much-needed supply of essential oxygen and blood to the body parts. While it is fashionable to talk about the benefits of the physical exercise on the heart and other body parts, we tend to overlook the master, i.e. the brain. The brain may be just 2% of our body weight, but it utilises 20% of our energy via blood and oxygen. It requires huge quantity of oxygen to function optimally. And physical activity ensures adequate supply of oxygen to the brain as well as all other body parts. In fact, it is a sort of health assurance. We seek health insurance to provide us monetary compensation for our maladies, but physical activity is like health insurance-cum-assurance that promises health benefits plus monetary savings, thanks to low medical expenses because of our wellness.

While retirement promotes inactive lifestyles, active career life offers an effective and involuntary mechanism to ensure adequate physical activity, which retards ageing. The effects of old age will catch up eventually, but it need not be a long and debilitating experience. But then, we tend to forget the maxim that we teach in schools, "Physical exercise makes us healthy, wealthy and wise."

Mental Activity

The physical health solely cannot be either endearing or enduring unless accompanied by the mental health. It is a common myth that our mental powers decline, as we grow older. The believers of this myth often support their contention by pointing out that our brain loses almost one gram per year, as we grow older. But then, the average human brain weighs about 1300 grams, encompassing a staggering 100 miles of blood vessels and 15 billion cells. Although, we know very little about the precise functioning of the brain, yet we know for sure that our lifestyle has a lot to do with our mental performance. To keep this work of art as polished as possible, we need to regularly exercise it particularly during later years. With adequate protective measures, we cannot just preserve our brainpower, but can also look forward to improve our brains as we age. Several studies suggest that mental activity is the key to overall good health. It also protects us against several old age diseases like Alzheimer, memory deterioration, dementia, mental derangement and the rest.

Besides, age is a state of mind. In fact, your enthusiasm matters. If it is accompanied with willingness to capitalise on your wisdom, the playing field is level. You can even count on your wisdom, enriched by myriad experiences, to provide you a winning edge at any age. Mentally active lifestyle enables you to optimally draw on your wisdom and experiences to take better, informed professional decisions.

Living an active lifestyle does not mean that you have to slog fifty hours a week. Even twenty hours will do you a world of good. And it does not mean you have to work daily. Working just three days a week is good enough to provide you optimal health benefits and improve your cognitive performance.

Biological Ageing

Chronological ageing denotes our age as a number, whereas biological ageing is indeed the gradual destruction of our body. A very common myth is that chronological and biological ageing happen in tandem. It is not true. By adapting an active and healthy lifestyle, we can delay the effects of ageing. It can certainly help us to moderate, if not control our biological ageing, which is the factual indicator of health. A scheduled work life can equip us, physiologically and psychologically, to ward off the ageing accelerators to enable us to put up a better show in this game of biological ageing.

What is more, we never know what the future holds for us. Scientists have recently found a naturally occurring substance, rapamycin, which has anti-ageing DNA, that is to say, it can slow or even stop the ageing process. And this discovery seems to be a science fact rather than a science fiction, as it significantly extends the life expectancy of animals in laboratory tests. Then again, Patricia Boyle, a neuropsychologist at Rush University Medical Centre, found that having a goal in life can help people live longer. Boyle found in a recent research experiment that older adults with a higher sense of purpose had about half the risk of dying during the follow up period as compared to people with a lower sense of purpose.

And the link between eating less and living longer is known since ages. Many studies have substantiated this premise that a calorie-restricted, optimal nutrition diet can significantly extend our lifespan. Furthermore, now the scientists have demonstrated that an animal can live up to 30% longer if its intake is cut down by 30% of its usual diet. In a human, that comes to more than 20 years of life. Scientists have also evidenced that a genetically modified mice can live twice. In fact, it is too soon to know the real impact of CRON-diet (Calorie Restriction with Optimal Nutrition) on human beings, but there is no doubt that our lifespan is increasing with better nutrition and advances in medical research. These scientific prospects apart, we can take for granted that a fulfilling and regulated work life can surely help us to retard the ageing process to quite some extent.

Creative Cravings

'Career success' is not complete if one does not experience fulfilment of her or his creative urges. One should not view old age as a period of decline. In fact, it offers an opportunity to attain one's goals and bring one's life to a satisfying and gratifying completion. Creative cravings provide a compelling motivation to avail the opportunity that retirement presents to fulfil the most cherished aspirations. This may be a chance to change 'career success' from what it is to what it ought to be.

Many of us always wanted to do something special, but could not afford to undertake because of the obligations of a formal work life and other duties. Retirement is the ideal time to look at unfulfilled ideas, plans and prospects. This is the right time to explore whether you can make a career out of your passion. Even if you are not looking for monetary rewards, you should exploit your creative cravings in a formal manner to get the real sense of fulfilment, besides other non-monetary benefits of a scheduled life.

Taxing your Mind

The age-old adage, "The more you use it, the sharper it gets" is very true in the context of the human mind. However, taxing your mind is not about unnecessarily straining your mind. It is more to do with sometimes engrossing your mental faculties in some higher-level brain tasks that require your absolute attention, but preferably have no monetary or personal consequences. By challenging your mind with such complex exercises, you can keep your mind agile and enhance its physiological functioning. Such exercises have the potential to provide a good mental workout, besides offering all the benefits of a dynamic meditation, especially when you enjoy doing these tasks. When it comes to utilising your mind, an active career life provides you many opportunities to use your mind and at times tax it too.

Forgetting

On the other hand, seniors should consciously develop the habit of overlooking frivolous details to keep their mind clutter free. At times, some people become forgetful during their sunset years partly because they ignore to clear their brains. They let superfluous information accumulate in their psyche leading to the overstuffing of their brains. As the old saying goes, "Our mind is like a drunken monkey that jumps from one thing to another without any rhyme or reason." With such a deluge of trivia in your brain, you cannot effectively indulge in quality brain work.

As you clear clutter and insignificant minutiae from your mind, your mind will be lighter and can carry out higher-level mental activities without any stress.

This way forgetting plays an important part in optimising the mental functioning. That is why taxing your mind and forgetting makes a potent combination to address the stress of working in later years. Therefore, you should consciously try to direct your attention only on issues that are more important and cultivate a habit of deliberately sidestepping trivia. You can develop your own filtering scheme to separate out trivial data and facts at the outset, and absorb only relevant and significant information. And you can seek a career where you are not just required to clutter your mind with irrelevant details, but have to manage higher-level intellectual functions, which will improve your performance, qualitatively as well as financially.

Financial Needs

The post-retirement life span is increasing steadily, thanks to the increasing longevity. But then, it makes financial planning difficult for many. Nowadays, one needs to provide for bread and butter for many-many more years after formal retirement. In order to provide sufficient funds for the post-retirement needs and desires, one has to consider many factors like health issues, household expenses, inflation, ever growing life expectancy and fluctuations in returns on investments. However, when one continues to work after formal retirement, these factors are surely taken care of considerably if not fully. Secondly, an active work life eases up financial anxieties by enabling the right frame of mind to handle the money matters more thoughtfully and thriftily.

Self-control

Being an experienced person, you might have been enforcing discipline for long. Perhaps now is the time to discipline yourself and be lenient with others. You need to keep in mind that moderation and balance are the key words to get the most out of your golden years. Meaningful ageing demands you to be adaptable, willing to change. You need to view the changed circumstances as an opportunity to exemplify self-discipline and virtuousness. This you can do by demonstrating balance and moderation in working, eating, exercising and all that.

This aspect may be demanding, especially for people who are inflexible and are not adept at taking the transition in the right perspective. They ignore this new opportunity which offers a new challenge to prove their mettle. Moreover, many people harbour false notions that retirement means freedom from work life, which they mistakenly take as drudgery. They fantasise that they can truly enjoy life when there is no work in life. This may be deceptively true in the short term, perhaps as a change. Shortly, they lose touch with the world of work, and they become outdated after a while. But they realise their predicament only when they reach the point of no return.

Given that self-regulation may not always work considering the vulnerabilities of human nature, we can depend on a career to provide us a framework to regulate our routine. An active work life also promotes balance in other areas of our life.

Maintaining Identity

In the absence of right retirement planning, we may have to experience a major change in our schedule after retirement. As we spend a large part of our day at our workplace, our identity is linked with our career. The thought of uncertain identity is frightening to most of us. And it often leads to upsetting the existing social and emotional equations. Besides, a regular routine is very important to give space to ourselves, which in turn helps to maintain healthy relations with all the near and dear ones. The ideal routine suggested for the mankind (and selectively for the womankind also) is to divide the day in three equal parts wherein two parts are allocated to sleeping and working, whereas the third part is kept open-ended at the discretion of the individual. Continuing your career not only offers a social identity, but also provides the benefits of a regular routine, socialising, variety in life and all that. Well-ordered work habits will safeguard you from the sense of disenchantment, which is a common side effect of the post-retirement phase. And it will serve the purpose if you engage yourself in a spiritual or other social activity to give back to the society. You can also pamper yourself in the luxury of your favourite leisure pursuits to maintain your schedule and social identity.

Analysing the Big Picture

The purpose of recapping the above-mentioned important factors is to enable you to capture the big picture of your golden years. Now, in the light of these factors, we proceed to analyse the big picture and assess your preparedness for the later years comprising the special third part of your mature life.

The following questions are configured to stimulate you with an eye to prepare you for the required groundwork for your post-retirement years. You need to write each question on a separate sheet of paper and scribble down as many answers as you can possibly think. Attempt to explore your answers from as many perspectives as possible. Here our objective is not just to find the best answer to your post-retirement issues, but also to immerse you in the process of creating a golden career vision for your silver years. However, the process can be an overwhelming experience for few vulnerable people. But perseverance is the key to make it work for you. This is essentially an engagement exercise that is intended to gauge as well as fortify your conviction to opt for a suitable post-retirement career. So, please bear in mind that the process is equally important, if not more than the outcome.

✓ Are you looking forward to retirement?

✓ How many post-retirement years do you guesstimate in the future?

✓ Do you appreciate the importance of a schedule and routine during sunset years?

✓ Are you dreading retirement? If your reply is yes, what are the reasons?

✓ Do you have a reliable career plan for the post-retirement years?

✓ How are you going to maintain your standard of living with increasing inflation and declining returns on investments?

✓ Have you assessed the implications if you outlive your investments?

✓ How you propose to constructively use your time in retirement?

✓ Have you clearly evaluated lifelong commitments such as health, finances, family, and fitness?

You are required to interpret and analyse these questions as well as their answers as a first step to your retirement planning. If you already have post-retirement career vision in place, these may perhaps indicate the extent of your preparedness. Brain storming over the above-mentioned factors is sure to provide you a direction as well as the requisite momentum to your retirement planning endeavours. You must make a note of the important pointers from the above exercise. These can help you immensely in organising your thoughts and developing the most pertinent career vision for your golden years.

Fortunately, more and more people are displaying strong urge to continue active work life even after formal retirement. They appreciate the benefits of working during golden years. And the age barrier does not deter willing people. They like to explore other lines of work to make the most of their skills and abilities. And they know that the new economy has many openings for the deserving people.

3

Planning Your Post-retirement Career

The process of creating career vision for golden years is not the same for everyone, because the reasons and conditions are different for each person. As far as post-retirement career planning is concerned, every individual has a unique profile due to different needs, preferences, qualifications, skills, experience and the like. It is neither feasible nor desirable to design a standard career plan for everyone. However, the following pointers are more or less common to all of you. They can help you to prepare well for the intended transition.

- ✓ Assess yourself
- ✓ Reflect on your goals
- ✓ Be realistic about your goals

✓ Match your interests

✓ Explore options

✓ Calculate your financial needs

✓ Stay positive

✓ Think yourself youthful

✓ Take time to contemplate

✓ Try out new career options

✓ Cope with the anxiety

✓ Be adaptable and tolerant

✓ Maintain your network

Our objective is to reacquaint you with your strengths and proficiencies so as to put you in a better position to envision a better career strategy resulting in a fitting and flexible career plan for your later years. This will provide you many useful insights to help you plan better for this transition. It is advisable to plan on your own or get yourself reasonably involved in the process of planning a great, fulfilling and rewarding career for your golden years. Even when you seek personalised professional advice, please do not restrict your participation to merely supplying the inputs for the creation of your plan.

Why People Lose Their Master's Touch After Retirement

It is important to note that many highly effective individuals lose their master's touch and flair when they take up their post-retirement careers. People invariably attribute this to the age factor, which may be partly true, particularly when the right attitude is lacking. However, moving into retirement with such misapprehensions can be intimidating for many people. Consequently, they loath to prime themselves to make good use of their skills in retirement and as such fall in the trap of retirement reticence. However, experts suggest three other reasons for this decline in performance – opting for inapt work, failure to manage change and time mismanagement. We will touch on the importance of choosing a right vocation and a positive and practical change strategy in the following sections. At this point, we should reflect on time management, which again becomes all-important at this stage of career.

Time management is not new to you, as you have been practising it throughout your career. And you know how to economise your time and follow a judicious approach to prioritise your to-do-list. Nevertheless, it has been observed that erroneous embedded perceptions of more than enough free time after retirement often leads to time mismanagement in the post-retirement phase. Besides, the ingrained certitude about the ability to manage time well often comes in the way of managing time optimally. In fact, time progressively becomes too valuable during later years and one must learn to manage it optimally.

But then, many seniors fail to benefit from the time-versus-outcome trade off. Time being at a premium for most people, they often require a system to evaluate and assign priorities to various activities on their agenda to maximise their output. But seniors do not get much help from the common urgent-important matrix wherein only one quadrangle out of four gets due priority. And the matrix routinely leads to non-performance in other three non-urgent and/or non-important areas until they turn into urgent and important thereby causing more unscheduled pressure on this limited resource. Further, compulsion to allocate all tasks in four segments often obfuscates the thinking process to prioritise the 'to-do-list' optimally and rationally.

You may fine-tune your own time management system to suit your current requirements. Remember you can multiply your throughput by making yourself conscious of each task's relative importance. And you can do just that with the following prioritisation system, which is a tried and trusted tool to multiply the productivity in value terms.

Schedule Prioritisation Template

This simple template helps you to objectively assign relative priorities to your to-do-list considering your defined preferences as well as the urgency factor. This is a very easy yet effective tool to optimise your productivity in an unbiased manner. This will not only unlock the door to increased productivity in your work life, but will also bring greater fulfilment and joy in your personal life because it effectively minimises the work related stress. The template can be created in many ways by incorporating as many factors as required. However, here we illustrate a basic version, which is good enough to meet the requirements of most people.

Directions:

→ List all your tasks in the first column of a spreadsheet/table.

→ In the second column, rate urgency of the task on a scale of 1 to 10 where 10 is the maximum urgency.

→ In the third column, rate significance of the task to your main driver A on a scale of 1 to 10 where 10 is the highest rating. Driver A is your prime motivator for your golden years' career.

→ In the fourth and fifth columns, rate significance of the task to your driver B and driver C (other dominant reasons persuading you to work besides driver A) on a scale of 1 to 5, where 5 is the highest rating.

→ Total all the scores for a particular task in the last column.

→ Sort all the tasks based on total scores to get your serialised priority list.

To-do-List (Tasks)	Urgency Factor	Driver A (Primary)	Driver B (Secondary)	Driver C (Secondary)	Total Score
Aaaab					
Bbbbc					
Ccccd					
Dddde					
Eeeef					
Ffffg					
Ggggh					
Hhhhi					
Iiiiiiiz					

You can very well prioritise your schedule yourself, but it is a better option to adapt a system wherein you just need to input your basic preferences, i.e., ratings to get your personalised agenda that enables you to robotically follow the priorities assigned by your system. It is a very simple method, yet it makes you highly effective and organised in your work life. Not only does it make you more productive, but it also makes you revalue the length of a certain length of time as per your yardstick.

In your schedule, you should allot some time for administrative and miscellaneous tasks as well as keep some flexibility to accommodate any unanticipated, urgent matters. You can afford to neglect or delegate the last few entries to free up your time that can be put to more productive, outcome-oriented use.

Being a mature person, you are conscious of the fact that you ought to adapt a selective approach to your various activities during golden years. Balance, moderation, limit and control are the key words to facilitate and strengthen your ability to deliver the output that capitalises on your skills and experience. You are also well aware that self-management is the key to success, particularly during later years. While managing our golden years on our own, occasionally overconfidence about our ability to manage these vulnerable factors becomes counterproductive to our objectives. Therefore, we ought to adapt a rational and realistic approach to realise our vision.

Predictably, some people solely looking to a life of

leisure may not like to change their definition of retirement. Perhaps, their hectic working life is responsible for their myopic thinking. But soon after retirement, they realise that a hectic work life is certainly better than a life full of leisure. Sooner or later, self-indulgence becomes bitter for them. But for now, such leisure-oriented, pleasure-seeking people may consider me somewhat biased on this topic. But I cannot help as my life's experiences and myriad examples persuade me to believe in this golden saying for golden years, "To a fool, old age is a bitter winter; to a wise man it is a golden time."

However, I believe that after a thorough analysis of various factors, you will agree with my firm view that it is desirable to continue work in one form or the other during golden years. This approach will help you to stay mentally and physically active, enjoy social interaction and secure your financial future. With some planning and enthusiasm, you can develop a new perception of sunset years that can provide you enough fuel for your forward journey for the rest of your life.

4

You Are Never Too Young To Retire

In general, early retirement refers to withdrawal from work before the mandatory retirement age. It can be availed at any age, but normally employed people consider it only after a tenure or age that qualifies them for the employer-provided retirement benefits. But nowadays people of any age are looking at it, because the needs and the options available today are far more stimulating than ever before. The option of early retirement attracts many people as it offers them an opportunity to make the most of their potential. They see it as a shortcut to realise their professional aspirations.

As is the case with other areas of life, our career life cannot always be evenly balanced. So, the thoughts of early retirement often cross the minds of most people while traversing ups and downs of work life. It is no longer unusual. And it is quite common in all the professions, even in the supposedly exciting professions. This trend is likely to gather momentum with the advent of knowledge economy and an enabling environment.

And the process of thinking over early retirement is not a bad idea because it invariably helps us to get the true picture of our professional life. And relating to our professional journey is always a good idea. So, let us explore the desirability and viability of early retirement in a dispassionate manner.

Why People Look At Early Retirement?

Unfortunately, most people, who consider early retirement, never aptly appreciate why they are mulling over it. They do not realise the seriousness of this decision. And often their decision is prompted by some immediate triggers. Even when they contemplate their compelling reasons to retire early, these are likely to be obvious, one-dimensional factors based on their limited understanding or lack of it. It is so because they tend to take a narrow and shallow view of their early retirement move. They even fail to examine the reasons, which prompted and influenced successful people who availed it to advance their career. That is why it is important to clearly understand your compelling reasons as well as appreciate the general triggers prompting people to opt for the early retirement. The early retirement triggers can be broadly grouped into two categories – personal and professional.

Common personal factors, which influence the early retirement decision, are family problems, health issues, children's education, working hours mismatch, family relocation and other personal reasons. In most of these cases, retirement planning entails more of financial and life planning issues rather than professional aspects. Even in such cases, people should strive to productively use their expertise and time. The misconception that work during sunset years was only meant for the needy class is surely fading away. Today, people want to be professionally active throughout their life. Individuals, who are mulling over early retirement to pursue leisure time activities or other social engagements, should also explore the ways to combine their interests within the framework of a formal routine of work life.

Deliberating on the personal issues is not only beyond the scope of this book, but we also believe that the intended readers are much more knowledgeable and wise to suitably deal with their personal issues. Besides, these personal issues vary significantly from person to person. But we would like to emphasise the importance of associating your family and friends in this important decision. As it is not always possible for a physician to rightly diagnose himself, likewise whenever you get overwhelmed with emotions or other personal factors while dealing with the early retirement dilemma, you should not hesitate to seek the help of your loved ones. In the extreme cases of indecisiveness, it is prudent to seek expert advice since this turning point is too important to sit by or take a wrong turn.

Professional reasons also induce many people to consider early retirement. Typically, people are very ambitious but, more often than not, their line of work curbs their aspirations. At times, professional reasons persuade them to exploit their skills and abilities in other work areas or work settings, which offer better incentives and growth prospects in addition to career continuity as long as they want.

Professional reasons can be grouped into external and individual factors, which can be further categorised as controllable and uncontrollable as well as positive and negative. While the positive factors encourage you to move on to achieve success and realise your cherished vision, the negative and often uncontrollable factors prod you to move out because of the adverse circumstances affecting you. Here are some common professional reasons.

> Sector specific problems due to economic recession

> Technological advances impacting the industry

> Organisation level downsizing

➢ Mismatch between job demands and personal skills

➢ Experiencing a career plateau

➢ Cravings for creative urges or challenges

➢ So called mid-life crisis instigating a change

➢ Unable to get along with seniors/colleagues

➢ Urge to leave the beaten track

➢ Self-pressure for professional achievement

➢ Dissatisfaction with the present work

➢ Desire for professional skills upgradation

➢ Frustration with the present work conditions

➢ Differences between groups such as young gang vs. old group

➢ Attraction to entrepreneurship or any other vocation

➢ Lack of job security or emotional stability

➢ Conflict with the organisational values, goals, policies

➢ Restricted financial growth

➢ Mismatch with the retirement vision

Often people explore early retirement because of job

dissatisfaction, which may be real or misperceived. More often than not, the root cause of the job dissatisfaction is attributable to the personal factors such as incompetence, mid-life crisis, health or emotional problems and the like. In such a case, perhaps you need to have a second look at your opinion after analysing the reasons. You should first try to deal with the situation wherein rectifying your weaknesses should get a priority. It is in your interest. However, when forces beyond your control are playing spoilsport, you can consider a change in the work settings instead of thinking about early retirement in the true sense. When the early retirement decision is basically based on where you want to be as compared to where you are and a proper transition plan is in place, it is definitely a positive reasoning and you are on the right track.

As is the case with any transition, this phase may also possibly be a period of confusion, stress, worries and uncertainties. A well-informed and well thought-out approach to manage this transition can mitigate if not eliminate the impact of the worrying factors. But then, many people boldly and sometimes blindly opt for the early retirement. When people take a badly informed decision to retire early and become so obsessed with the process of implementing it, they do not realise that a plan that is born out of ignorance is also bound by the ignorance. Hence, it is advisable to check again the decision before proceeding further.

Are You Really Ready To Take Early Retirement?

It is important to examine your awareness and readiness for this transition before we discuss common positive and negative aspects of early retirement. So, you should first seek answers to the pertinent questions from your conscious and subconscious mind before assigning these to the tests of worldly wisdom. You need to unambiguously find out why you want to retire early. What is attracting you towards early retirement? Are you fully aware of the long-term implications? Are you emotionally and financially prepared for this transition? Questions abound. But these should not be construed as simple questions seeking straight answers.

You have to be doubly sure that you really want early retirement before you take the plunge. You are likely to take the right decision only when you clearly figure out whether the early retirement will serve your objectives or not. Brainstorming over the following exploratory questions will further give you some valuable insights to decide whether the early retirement is right for you.

✓ How much capital do you reckon is sufficient to opt for the early retirement?

✓ Are you emotionally and professionally ready to do something different in the retirement phase?

✓ What is the level of satisfaction in your present job?

✓ Do you get excited or weary with the thought of early retirement?

✓ What are your plans if you outlive your retirement reserves?

✓ Do you know the career field well that you wish to pursue after retirement?

✓ Do you have adequate resources to meet your family responsibilities?

✓ Have you discussed and taken the opinion of your family members?

✓ Have you done your groundwork for the golden years? Are your future plans ready and practical?

✓ Are your plans holistic in nature or just career-centric/self-centric?

✓ Do you have the requisite staying power and energy to achieve what you desire?

✓ Do you really want to be your own boss to tap your knowledge, skills and creativity? Or is it just that you want to make the transition from bossed to boss?

✓ Do you have the requisite mindset to diligently pursue your prospective course?

✓ Do you have what it takes to make this transition successful?

If you are not entirely satisfied with your answers, perhaps you are overlooking the necessary groundwork and contemplating the early retirement hastily. Remember once announced, it is awkward to 'unannounce' your retirement. That is why you need to prepare yourself adequately so that you can confidently navigate this important turning point of your career. You should focus on the realistic roadblocks accentuated by the above brainstorming exercise in order to overcome them or find the ways to sidestep them. Bear in mind that getting early retirement to switch to your dream career can be a truly interesting and rewarding proposition only if you have created a good and workable roadmap after examining the above-mentioned points.

After examining your personal issues, we take up some important and universally relevant positive and negative factors of the early retirement. These pros and cons along with your personal issues present all the pieces of the early retirement jigsaw puzzle. All these parameters will help you view the complete picture and take an informed decision.

Early Retirement Pros:

+ Unleash your potential: When you aspire to use your creative potential in the golden years, early retirement puts you in an advantageous position by providing you the first mover advantage. And it is always better to start your new occupation as early as possible so that you have an established career by the conventional retirement age. It is much easier to continue an established career during golden years than starting a new one.

+ Better adaptability to a new career: Early retirement enables you to become habituated to your new career relatively at a younger age. You can make better use of your energy and skills to establish in your new career. You need not endure the work demands of a start-up or a new job during your golden years. Your mind and body will also get used to your new work life by the standard retirement age.

+ Financial rewards: More and more people are flirting with the idea of early retirement mainly because of its potential to offer greater financial rewards in the long run. They appreciate that life expectancy is going up and their savings and retirement benefits are not likely to keep pace with the inflation owing to the dwindling returns on the financial investments. They seek to overcome this financial dilemma by aiming at superior financial reimbursement for their skills over an extended period of time.

+ Long-term career creation: Early retirement can enable you to create a career wherein you can continue to work as long as you deem fit. It also provides you flexibility on many other counts like working hours, type and scale of work, remote management of work, etcetera. Moreover, when you establish a business, you create a regular source of income for your loved ones; besides, you will leave a mark of your expertise that will inspire them forever.

+ Your own initiative: When you choose early retirement to pursue a work line, it is your initiative. It gives you a sense of purpose that is likely to be diluted when you undertake the same work line after retirement age. When you start something voluntarily and purposely, it gives you ample motivation and drive to succeed. There is surely a big difference between choosing the path and tagging along the beaten path.

Early Retirement Cons:

- Stability: When you are settled in your job, you experience a sense of security that you are not likely to get in any new career or after retirement. Reliability of a well-established career cannot be compared with the uncertainties of any new situation, where many negatives usually crop up from nowhere after you take the plunge. In an established career, you are quite insulated from the vagaries of the uncertain and competitive world of work.

- Financial security: After working for so many years, one becomes used to the monthly cheque, and thus may not appreciate its importance fully as it is taken for granted. In addition to the monthly cheque, one gets many perquisites which come only as long as one is employed. But we feel the real pinch when we have to dig into our savings to meet our expenses.

- Established schedule: When you follow an established schedule continuously for a long period, not only your mind and body become habituated to it but your loved ones also get used to it. Any disruption in your set schedule may possibly cause discomfort to you and to those around you, especially when you have voluntarily opted for it. Set schedule has its own advantages that should not be overlooked. It provides you mental and physical activity without causing undue strain. And it leaves little or no time for unhealthy lifestyle.

- Time to prime yourself: In case the main purpose of considering early retirement is to start a career that you can continue during sunset years, it may perhaps be a better option to take your own time to reflect on your proposed career while continuing in the present employment. You can use this time to explore the alternatives as well as prime yourself properly to ensure a better outcome from your venture. This investment of time and energy can save you from committing costly mistakes at the implementation stage when you also have to fend for yourself and your dependant family members. You can also make use of the time until the age of formal retirement to complete groundwork and develop your network so as to facilitate a smooth transition.

How to Decide

After evaluating the above-mentioned benefits and drawbacks along with other personal issues, it can be an overwhelming experience for any normal person to take a final call. It is not easy to take a dispassionate decision, particularly in the absence of any decision-making framework. Consequently, it often leads to procrastination, and in many cases missing the opportunity. But then, we can always explore some decision-making techniques to take an unbiased and pragmatic decision even under such an involved situation. One such technique is force field analysis pioneered by Kurt Lewin. This remarkable technique gives the idea to develop a decision making model for the early retirement predicament. Here, we briefly discuss this objective and appropriate technique to sort out the dilemma of taking a decision for or against the early retirement option.

In our context, the force field analysis provides a quantifiable qualitative as well as quantitative structure to evaluate the positive and negative forces that influence a change decision. This technique defines pros as driving forces that will support change, i.e., in favour of early retirement. And cons are defined as restraining forces that oppose the change, i.e., against early retirement. It is really an effective technique as it offers a 360-degree view by depicting all the relevant pros and cons in an objective manner. To elucidate this technique, here I am illustrating it with some modifications so that a clear-cut direction emerges as the outcome of this exercise.

Creating Force Field Analysis:

→ Describe the proposal, i.e. whether to opt for early retirement or not.

→ Think and list all the pros, i.e. driving forces in left side of the table as depicted. Keep your mind on the left side of the table only and allot a score to each force i.e. pros on a scale of 1 to 5 where 1 is weakest and 5 is strongest.

→ Think and list all the cons, i.e. restraining forces in the right side of the table. Focus on the right side of the table only and allot a score to each force, i.e. cons on a scale of 1 to 5 where 1 is weakest and 5 is strongest.

→ Draw arrows in proportion to the scores pointing towards right for pros, i.e. factors supporting early retirement.

→ Draw arrows proportionate to the score pointing towards left for cons, i.e. factors opposing early retirement.

→ Calculate the total score of driving and restraining forces at the corresponding side at the bottom of the table.

→ You may go ahead with the decision if driving forces outnumber restraining forces by a decent margin.

Driving Forces	Early Retirement? YES NO		Restraining Forces
Utilise unused potential → → → →	4	3	Financial security ← ← ←
Lasting career continuity → → →	3	3	Need time to reflect ← ← ←
Financial rewards → → →	3	3	Career Stability ← ← ←
Right age to start → →	2	2	Social links @ work ← ←
Right time → →	2		
Job dissatisfaction → →	2		
Right opportunity → →	2		
TOTAL +	18 →	←11	TOTAL -
Decision:	+7 In Favour		

Perhaps, you were aware of this decision, but it becomes simpler to navigate when it is objectively given in the black and white. And when the decision derived from the above analysis is not to your liking, you may brainstorm over the ways to boost up the score of driving forces and minimise the influence of restraining forces or vice-versa in order to maximise the chances of your desired outcome. It provides you the right perspective and direction as well as an opportunity to make it feasible in the near future. Our objective is not to project any direction as a panacea for all the post-retirement challenges, but just to give a ringside view of the post-retirement challenges to enable the learned readers to take a well-informed and well-reasoned decision.

Finally, yet importantly, no technique or advice can substitute your own view of the decision considering your personal parameters. And you must remember that while it can open new doors of personal growth and future opportunities, it is also likely to close many doors to the past. Therefore, you must try to ensure that your decision is consistent with your needs and not just your wants. Ideally, you should aspire to strike the right balance.

5

What Do You Really Want From Your Career

Retirement is never just a retirement, but also a repository of our insecurities, anxieties, worries, and even sense of worthlessness. And it is not just the financial insecurity, which leads to all these concerns. Many people fail to acknowledge these non-financial apprehensions, which may manifest or not. They live with the delusion that future will take care of itself. So, they procrastinate their future planning for golden years even though they are aware of the advantages it offers.

Often their feeble argument for this apathy is that retirement is the time for liberty. Liberty to relax, enjoy life and undertake leisure pursuits that they could not afford while working. It sounds good in theory. In real life, worldly pleasures alone cannot ensure happiness for long. At best, they can present an interim illusion of happiness.

Besides, there is an identity angle to the retirement. Our identity is usually an extension of our career. It may not be so obvious before retirement, but it slowly and surely sinks in after retirement. But then, if we appreciate this angle and make appropriate plans to address this issue, we may never experience the 'identity dilution'– a common side effect of retirement.

Wise people choose the right way to overcome this tricky situation by continuing their work life well beyond the usual retirement age. Given that most experts on ageing recommend active lifestyle to improve quality of life in later years, it makes good sense to continue working or gradually reduce professional activities. Nowadays more and more people are heeding to this advice, perhaps in their own style.

The years after the conventional retirement age cover about one-third time of our life. These golden years can be the most productive years of your life after acquiring knowledge and experience in the first two-thirds of your life. All you need to do is to make the right moves now to get the optimal benefit from your later years. So, do not waste time now in doubts and fears; invest some time in planning your next career move, well assured that this will be the best preparation for your golden years. You can surely benefit by deploying your skills, expertise and wisdom in many intellectually stimulating and financially rewarding vocations. When the time for real retirement comes, you can contentedly apply the brakes on your successful and extended career journey. You owe it to yourself, your family and the society to make the best use of your abilities.

Career Selection Criteria

By now, it may not be very difficult to decide whether you should work during golden years or not. But, you may have to take into account several factors to decide how you should choose your career for the golden years. While choosing your career for the later years, it is very important that first you identify your main drivers that inspire you towards a post-retirement career. Being an experienced and mature person, you ought to be quite familiar with general as well as your specific drivers that influence your career decisions. Remember, these pointers are equally relevant while choosing a worthwhile post-retirement career. Now you can use the following three simple steps to finalise your deciding drivers, which will enable you to choose a compatible career.

1. Take a sheet of paper and divide it into two columns. In the first column, write three most important factors directing you to a post-retirement career. In the second column, you have to justify your factors by writing reasons

supporting the corresponding factor. Now, set timer for ten minutes for the first factor. Scribble down your arguments as fast as you can. It would be better if you complete this exercise without a pause. Repeat the exercise for the second and third factors.

2. Next day take a copy of the list and try to analyse each factor and its justifications for thirty minutes– as a critic.

3. After a few days or a week, take both the lists and brainstorm over each factor and related reasons. Try to add/delete/modify as much as you want in order to make a final list of prime motivators with their justifications. When the final list is ready, devote half an hour to mentally soak up the main reasons that prompt you to seek a post-retirement career.

In addition to these prime motivators, you should also look for the following imperative qualities in your preferred career.

- ✔ Conviction in the mission and vision of the endeavour

- ✔ An opportunity to make a genuine and good contribution

- ✔ Likely intellectual stimulation and mental growth

- ✔ A chance to draw on your expertise
- ✔ An opportunity to stay up to date with the latest in the field
- ✔ Work gratification and enjoyment
- ✔ Sense of accomplishment

Appropriate Categories of Careers

After appreciating the importance of continuing your career in retirement and acquainting yourself with your prime drivers, you are all set to explore the suitable categories of careers for your golden years.

People often blame the lack of suitable opportunities for retirees for not having a retirement career plan in place. And their reluctance to look beyond the obvious is understandable considering their long experience. But then, your decision to select a particular field or career should not be a compulsive or impulsive decision.

We are supposed to choose our calling based on our profile, but we should also be receptive to other viable options at the exploration stage. We need to spend some time in a careful, systematic search so that finally we can opt for an apt opportunity. And we should not lose our nerves in the process and take up any vocation that comes to our mind. In order to succeed, we ought to first concentrate on doing the right things, then on doing things right. Here we are outlining a few pertinent categories of careers and hope one of these can make your golden years a truly golden era.

Continue Old Career

The charm of the known is strong, and addictive. Therefore, this is the obvious choice of many people. After diligently working for a very long period, it may be unnerving proposition for many people to think about other careers. Considering the basic human nature, the feeling is natural. In addition, people are likely to have better network and knowledge about right opportunities in their field. But to make an impact, you have to maintain your proficiency level and keep yourself abreast of the latest in your field.

Self-employment in Your Preferred Field

At this stage of career, many people have an aversion to be subordinated to the people who are less qualified and/or experienced as compared to them. As the seniors make transition from bossed to boss, they can look forward to many other incentives and flexibilities offered by the self-employment. It can offer flexible schedule, financial incentives and intellectually rewarding work. It suits senior people well since they have acquired many transferable skills and abilities during their career, which they can put to good use in many ways and many areas on a freelance basis.

Promote your Hobby as your Career

People who are passionate about any pursuit can seriously consider making a career out of that. Apparently, this is the best possible career category given that you can enjoy your hobby as well as make money out of it. But, it is important to check whether it will fulfil all your needs and wants in the long run. Remember that your hobbies and interests change over a period. And then going overboard is a common pitfall of this category. So, you may perhaps pick only those assignments that you really like in order to reasonably regulate your work schedule. It will give you enough time for other personal priorities as well as keep your interest alive. However, you need to adapt a professional approach in your endeavour not only to create a successful business from your hobby, but also to derive all the benefits of a scheduled work life.

Shift to a New Career Field

If your field does not excite you anymore or you are just fed up with the work environment, you may explore employment in a different field. As many skills are easily transferable to many other professions, many people prefer to change career field to fulfil their hankering need to do something new. After working for a long period, some people find their career line somewhat monotonous and tedious work. If you find your current work repetitive and boring, you may look at other careers which can provide you enough opportunities to exploit your true potential.

However, you can explore a suitable and fitting job in other fields of your choice to savour the experience of working in a new exciting field. But, before opting for a job in a new career field, you need to clarify your skills and interests before making up your mind about the job so that you can truly enjoy your career during your silver years.

Start a Business

If you want to be your own boss, stay active, enjoy freedom and test your entrepreneurial skills, you may think about starting a small (or big) business. Here stakes are likely to be much higher as compared to other career categories. So are the rewards. Massive fortunes of wealthy people are not amassed through service, but through entrepreneurship. Further, your business gives you the liberty to balance career with family and other responsibilities. If you have reasonably provided for all your financial needs until the break-even point of the proposed venture and have genuine conviction in your concept, you may examine this option at any age. First step is to explore the market for your output and ascertain the demand vs supply equation by conducting a market research in an objective manner. Market analysis of your product and/or service is very important to assess the viability of your idea.

Volunteer Yourself

If you belong to the fortunate few who do not have financial concerns and have the strong urge to give back something to the society, volunteer work can be truly gratifying for you. Many people prefer to live modestly in retirement and volunteer their time to social, cultural or environmental projects in their local communities. You can reconfirm what your endearing and enduring passions are and take up some social work related to these passions in a formal manner. You should consider only such opportunities which are in harmony with your interests and aspirations. Such a work will keep you constructively engaged to make your golden years truly gratifying.

What Do You Want From Your Career

Before exploring specific career options, it would be helpful to look at some other aspects about you and your career experiences. It will facilitate intelligent scanning of other occupations. Brainstorming over the following common questions will stimulate your thinking and help you to take a well thought-out decision.

> ➢ Am I interested in a job or self-employment?

➤ Am I seeking diversity & challenge or stability & security?

➤ Am I open to a career in a new but promising field?

➤ Am I looking for standard work hours or flexible timings?

➤ Do I aspire to extend my career life as long as possible?

➤ Do I prefer to work from home?

➤ Am I willing to relocate?

➤ Am I comfortable with the competition?

➤ Major experiences I liked from the present and previous jobs.

➤ Major experiences I disliked from the present and previous jobs.

➤ The level of autonomy and creativity I need to experience the career bliss.

➤ How important are the financial rewards to me?

➤ What is the need and importance of critical thinking or intellectual stimulation for me?

➤ Do I clearly understand my career orbit and my present placement in that?

Before contemplating a career shift, it is important to look at all worthy occupations that are particularly suitable for you. This exercise can reveal some careers that you may not have thought about earlier. What's more, you will find that experience and skills acquired by you are easily transferable to many such careers in various fields and as such, you are already eligible for these careers. However, it is important that you only consider careers that are in demand and complement your retirement vision.

6

108 Post-Retirement Careers

After you recognise what truly matters to you, it is easy to focus on what you really want to do. Now you are in a position to figure out how you should use your existing skills and talents in order to experience fulfilment, success and a joyous life. And while doing so, remember that the objective is to make the most of your retirement years and reward yourself for your accomplishments over the years.

Some of the probable careers suitable for seniors are outlined hereunder. Please do not restrict your career orbit to this list. This is just to stir up your thinking and acquaint you with some interesting career options. When you look around and search, you can also discover some interesting careers befitting your post-retirement plan. Such careers can be more appropriate, as they emerge from within you and invariably supported by the favourable external factors. But remember that you have to thoroughly research any career option that stimulates you and appears to be your dream vocation. Here is a brief explanation of the Career Options Catalogue.

➢ Column 1 depicts a brief description of Designation/ Occupation.

➢ Column 2 shows suitability of a career in the job mode (J) or as a self-employed enterprise (S). The occupations suitable for both the modes are expressed as either J/S or S/J wherein first letter indicates somewhat better scope than the next letter.

➢ Column 3 shows the typical working hours for a career. R and F indicate a career's suitability for Regular/specific hours or Flexible hours respectively.

➢ Column 4 depicts the outlook for the relevant career on a scale of A to E where A points to the best outlook and E refers to the bleak outlook. These are broad indicators, which may vary from place to place depending on the current demand and supply situation of the talent in the region and/or occupation.

➢ Column 5 shows the expected requirement of new skills, which are obligatory in order to adeptly undertake the respective career, on a scale of 1 (negligible) to 5 (substantial).

Remember, awareness of the suitable careers makes it easier for you to explore viable options you might not have been able to scan before. It helps you to envision careers based on your core strengths, and thus can help you to realise your vision for the golden years.

Some vocations are more appropriate for seniors considering their different needs and preferences. This aspect is particularly important and relevant for retiring people since they possess a knowledge based skills-set in addition to other administrative qualities. After a lifetime of working, they usually develop a different type of mindset that makes them more suitable for some careers and not so suitable for others. Here are some careers which are suitable for retiring individuals.

The Career Options Catalogue

Designation/ Occupation	Career Mode	Working Hours	Future Outlook	New Skills
Financial Planner	S/J	R/F	A	4
Children's Party Planner	S	F	B	1
Marriage Counsellor	S	F/R	B	2
Career Planning Counsellor	S/J	R/F	B	3
Dance/Music Trainer	S/J	R/F	C	1/4
Content/Blog Writer	S/J	F/R	B	2/4
Public Relations- Coordinator	J/S	R/F	C	2
Customer Services Provider	J/S	R/F	C	2
Consultant-Relationships	S	F	B	3
Games, Software Creator or Tester	S/J	F/R	C	4

Designation/ Occupation	Career Mode	Working Hours	Future Outlook	New Skills
Educational Products Demonstrator	S/J	F/R	C	2
Motivational Speaker	S	F	C	3
Workshop Presenter	S	F	C	2
Library or Museum Guide	J/S	R/F	D	3
Foreign Education Consultant	S/J	F/R	C	3
Newspaper/Magazine Reporter/Editor	J/S	R/F	C	3
Administrative Officer	J	R	C	3
Insurance Consultant	S/J	F/R	B	4
Procurement Specialist/ Agent	J/S	R/F	C	4
Writer- Booklets & Magazine Articles	S	F	B	2/4
Human Resources Expert	S/J	R/F	B	3
Manufacturer's Sales Representative	S/J	F/R	D	2
Market Researcher/Surveyor	J/S	R/F	B	2
Business Amenities Provider	S	R/F	A	2
Wedding Planner/Services	S	F	C	2
Recording /Dubbing Professional	S	F	C	3

Designation/ Occupation	Career Mode	Working Hours	Future Outlook	New Skills
Reception/Conference Organiser	S/J	F/R	B	2
Event Planner/Coordinator	S	F	C	3
Dance Therapist	S	F	C	2/4
Occupation Counsellor	S/J	F/R	B	3
Fashion Consultant	S	F	B	3
Graphic Designer/Animator	J/S	R/F	B	1/5
House Keeping Services/ Advisor	S	F/R	C	3
Office/Home Hygienist	S/J	F/R	B	2
Purchase Coordinator	J/S	R/F	C	3
Interpreter / Translator	J/S	R/F	C	2/5
Interior Designer/Re-designer	S/J	F/R	C	3
Journalist-General/Domain Specialist	J/S	R/F	C	3
Logistics Expert	S/J	R/F	C	4
Music Trainer/Therapist	S/J	R/F	C	2/5
Dietician/Nutritionist	S/J	F/R	C	2
Safety Expert	J/S	R/F	C	2
Computer Security Expert	S/J	F/R	B	5
Travel Planner	S	F	C	2

Designation/ Occupation	Career Mode	Working Hours	Future Outlook	New Skills
Transportation Services	S	R/F	C	3
Records Administrator	J	R	D	2
Recreational Therapist/Services	S	R/F	B	2
Restaurant Manager	J	R	B	2
Retailer- Innovative Products	S/J	R	C	2
Sales & Marketing	J/S	R/F	C	3
Scholastic Counsellor	S	F/R	B	2
Placement Coordinator	S/J	F/R	B	2
Literary Agent	S	F	B	3
Relationship Counsellor	S/J	R/F	A	3
Yoga / Aerobics Instructor	S/J	F/R	B	3
Landscaping Services/ Expert	S	F	B	3
Theme Party Organiser	S	F	B	2
Warehousing /Storage Services	S/J	R/F	C	3
Cosmetic & Personal Care Consultant	S	F	C	2
Residential Complex Upkeep	S/J	R/F	D	3
Fitness & Sports Centre	S/J	F	C	2
Credentials Verification Services	S	F	B	3

Designation/ Occupation	Career Mode	Working Hours	Future Outlook	New Skills
Security Needs Appraiser	S	F	B	3
Fleet &/or Armoured Car Services	S/J	R/F	C	2
Equipment Maintenance Services	S	F/R	D	4
Exhibition Organiser	S	F	C	3
Home Health Care Services	S	F	C	2
Freelance Artist / Performer	S	F	D	2/5
Decorating Services	S	F/R	B	2
Florist – Chain/ Online	S	F	C	2
Compatibility Assessor	S	F	A	3
Marriage Facilitator	S	F	B	2
Distribution Services	S	R/F	C	3
Pet Grooming Services	S	F	C	3
Animals Warden/ Crèche	S	R	C	3
Advertising Stuff Designer	S/J	F/R	C	4
Recycling Specialist	S	F	B	3
Customer Care Services	J/S	R/F	C	2
News Analyst/ Media Surveyor	S/J	F/R	B	3
Real Estate Analyst	S/J	R/F	B	4

Designation/ Occupation	Career Mode	Working Hours	Future Outlook	New Skills
Sports Academy	S	F/R	C	3
Business Development Services	J/S	R/F	B	3
Business Facilities Provider	S	F	C	2
Training Needs Assessor	S	R/F	B	4
Theme Crèche	S	F/R	B	2
Computer Instructor	J/S	R/F	B	1/4
Language Specialist/Services	S/J	F/R	C	1/4
Fund Raiser	S	F	D	2
Food Services	S	R/F	C	1
Speech Writer	S	F	B	2/4
Consultant- Kids Issues	S	R/F	B	3
Health Resort/Centre	J/S	R/F	C	2
Scholastic Publisher	S	R/F	C	3
Branch Office Services	S/J	R	C	2
Personal Coach	S/J	F/R	B	1
Baby Care Counselling	S	F	B	3
Art Gallery Owner/Manager	S/J	R/F	B	2/3
Books/ Periodicals Critic	S	F	B	4
Logo, Emblem etc. Designer	S/J	F/R	C	2/4
Speech Therapist	S	F	C	3

Designation/ Occupation	Career Mode	Working Hours	Future Outlook	New Skills
Tours Planner/Organiser	S/J	F/R	D	3
Uniforms Designer	S	F	C	2
Investment Advisor	S/J	F/R	A	4
Culture Boutiques	S	F	B	3
Health/ Fitness Specialist	S/J	F/R	C	2
Trends Miner	S/J	F/R	C	2
Divorce Planner/ Facilitator	S	F	B	3
Motivational Interviewer	S/J	F/R	B	4

Now we briefly look into how one can impetuously trim down the probable careers list i.e. careers which interest you and match your retirement vision. Here we intend to illustrate how one can subjectively explore a few selected careers before objectively picking out the best career, which invariably calls for a detailed examination. For a simple illustration, here we take the first three above-mentioned options as your preferred careers choices.

Financial Planner

While practising financial planning for the golden years or other goals, many people develop a liking to this field, as money management has always been their forte and passion. Number crunching, analysis and money management aspects of this career give them the craved feeling of excitement, which they never savoured in their career. Being swift learners, they pick up a lot of knowledge about this field for their use, perhaps in an informal manner. This fondness can convince them to explore this line as their career as well as a leisure pursuit that can result in indirect and direct financial rewards.

Children's Party Planner

This career is ideally suited for people who are looking at a freelance career wherein they get a chance to be with children. For some individuals, the company of children is probably the main driver as they really miss it. They may not be interested in financial rewards, but people, who are adept at event organising, bulk buying and social skills, can gain a lot from this seemingly smallish service, even if they charge less than the market rates for their service. This can be a win-win situation for all the parties involved.

Marriage Counsellor

The typical work life involves a lot of social interaction. After devoting their lifetime to the world of work, many people become habituated to the social aspects of it. Behavioural analysis is their inherent strength and human beings are their favourite subjects. Besides, they invariably miss the human interaction in retirement. Secondly, their all-round extensive experience makes them proficient in judging people. After dealing with and training so many people, they often have a better understanding of the emotional needs and social underpinnings of people. And most people are good at transforming reticent wannabes to receptive partners. These factors give them the competitive edge to offer a better premarital service to assess the all-important compatibility factor and other behavioural aspects to ensure a successful marriage. They may not rake in megabucks initially, but can definitely leave an impact on the field by substantially improving the success rate of marriages, wherein today's marriage counsellors have as dismal record as self-styled soothsayers.

Finalising Your Retirement Career

Next step is to analyse the short listed options in an objective manner to finalise the most suitable career. You can assign maximum marks to your prime drivers and other relevant factors depending on their significance in your life. Then you can give marks to these factors for each career option. While allocating marks, you must bear in mind the relative merit of each option as compared to others. By comparing the total score of various options, you will get an unbiased clue to your future calling. Here is a hypothetical illustration to clarify the concept. You can modify this table to suit your requirements.

Comparing Probable Careers

Deciding Factors	Maximum Score	Career A	Career B	Career C
Future Outlook				
Financial Rewards				
Job/Freelance Work				
Mandatory Skills				
Work Timings				
...				
....				
Personal reason 1				
Personal reason 2				
Personal reason 3				
...				
....				
Total				

New Beginning

Thanks to today's ever-growing economy, many organisations appreciate the value of veterans' skill sets. And their ability to learn and grasp swiftly makes them a much sought after category of contenders in many vocations. Also, their experience and role as a disciplinarian has many takers. Yet, seniors do not find enough opportunities at the top side of the career pyramid. They are often sidetracked for the top positions primarily because the veterans are used to a typical functioning style, a more directive command-and-control style. Some seniors acquire this functioning style while exercising their authority in their long career. But then, today's business world generally practices a somewhat different work style; a more democratic, flexible and sharing control type of attitude to working. However, people can easily climb the ladder from demanding, monotonous careers to the prime careers with a little change in the attitude and a proper balancing to get the best of both work styles.

You are supposed to follow a somewhat different set of rules during post-retirement phase if you want to achieve your golden years' vision. This is especially important for people opting for a career in other fields. So, whatever vocation you choose, you must try to adapt to the change gracefully and make the most of this new beginning. Here are some pertinent pointers to help you secure a successful transition to your second beginning.

- ✓ Have conviction in your vision and resulting goals
- ✓ Rely on your abilities and practice 'can-do' attitude
- ✓ Be accountable to yourself and your vision
- ✓ Maintain self-respect at any cost
- ✓ Be optimistic and try to give your best
- ✓ Avoid complaining and blaming
- ✓ Continue to learn and watch trends in the field
- ✓ Avert self-obsolescence by all means
- ✓ Avoid self-justification attitude
- ✓ Show mature leadership
- ✓ Review old traditions. Don't stick to old practices.
- ✓ Manage time prudently
- ✓ Periodically compare with achievers
- ✓ Lead from your strengths. Try to exploit your speciality
- ✓ Welcome change and face reality
- ✓ Be humble and flexible

No one can be hundred percent sure that a new vocation can fulfil her or his retirement vision until she/he gets hands-on experience in that field. However, the process of career planning steers you in the right direction to improve your chances of success and prevent you from taking detrimental steps. And wisely planning your retirement career will ensure that you will not only live healthier and productive life, but also reap all the benefits you envisioned from your career. Having a clear vision for future and drawing optimally on your faculties are the keys to realise your vision. As you undertake your post-retirement career, let me urge you to take it as earnestly as you took your first career.

Golden years beckon you to allow your imagination to flourish, creativity to flower.

7

Retirement Reckonings: Giving Meaning To The Means

Retirement is a scary prospect for some people, especially when they think about the absence of monthly remuneration. With increasing lifespan, often retirement reserves comprising of both personal savings and retirement benefits are not enough for retirement, particularly when one is not sure about the post-retirement period one has to brave out on these savings. People are realising the need to be financially independent even after retirement, as they do not expect the government or others to bear the burden of their old age.

We have already emphasised a great deal on the health and social consequences of retirement deliberately skipping the financial aspects. The objective was just to trigger a healthy discussion on the relatively inconspicuous but equally important themes, which are often overlooked while attending to the more glorified and commercial theme, namely, financial planning for retirement. We live in a world where financial aspects of retirement are enthroned, and health, professional and social aspects are often subordinated. In fact, people often consider retirement planning as just planning finances for retirement. The intention was not to undermine the importance of financial aspects but to reinforce it.

Moreover, our financial health and physical health are mutually dependent and both enhance our life, and quality of our life. There is no contradiction between the two. Each gives valuable support to the other. So we need to accord equal priority to the both, as we cannot enjoy money without health or health without money.

Most senior readers are likely to be in good shape to take care of their financial concerns of the golden years. Yet, the financial planning for retirement is not as simple and clear-cut exercise as often made out by the vested interests. It can be a simple exercise but for numerous variables working waveringly. Many variables are external factors, i.e., factors beyond your control and hence cannot be accurately projected for future planning. Can you forecast rate of return on your investments after a decade? Can you predict fuel prices for the next year? Can you foresee health problems as well as related expenses after a decade or two? Can you foretell inflation rate for the next five years? Questions abound with no concrete solutions.

Just consider the consequences of price increases on your living expenses at various inflation rates. When inflation goes up, it does not mean returns on your market instruments will also go up. Returns on your market investments may possibly go down resulting in a double whack. Can you reasonably forecast your cost of living when you are 80 years old? The following table attempts to explore the impact of inflation on living expenses in percentage terms by considering inflation at 4% and 8%.

Consequences of Inflation on Retirees

Retirement Age	% Increase in cost of living by age 80	
Years	Inflation @ 4%	Inflation @ 8%
50	224	906
55	167	585
60	119	366
65	80	217

With just a few percentage points variation in one variable, i.e. inflation, your retirement budget may possibly go in for a toss. You may wonder what is the use of a comprehensive plan when we cannot predict the basic factors correctly. Perhaps you are right. But then, we know the statistically proven fact that travelling is one of the biggest risk factors, yet we cannot and do not give up travelling. However, we strive to make our travels as risk-free as possible.

I do not want to depict a gloomy picture. What I am emphasising is that it is an uncertain picture where one cannot be at ease by superficially balancing the retirement needs with the retirement reserves. I just intend to give a 360 degrees view of the retirement planning. This you may not get from your financial advisor, as s/he may perhaps like to skip some points that are counterproductive to her/his business interests. No wonder financial services are big business and are getting more and more profitable, often at the expense of gullible investors who misguidedly extrapolate trends.

However, one need not lose motivation because the doers can always find a way out, as we shall discuss shortly. Besides, in actuality, many negative and positive factors often counteract one another and the net negative impact, if any, is likely to be marginal. What is more, we tend to habituate ourselves to the present and blank out the distant time, which minimises the psychological impact of negatives enabling us to harness the positives.

In view of the many indeterminate factors at play, financial planning for retirement may be a challenging task but its importance cannot be overlooked. Developing a financial plan is imperative to understand our preparedness for the sunset years. The golden years can be a time of enjoyment, or the beginning of a nightmare, depending on the adequacy of our financial preparedness for the post-retirement period.

A recent study by HSBC found that people who planned for retirement had five times the assets of those who did not. Our retirement plan provides us a framework that shows us the direction and the way forward to secure our financial future. The benefits of financial planning for later years outweigh the uncertainties and challenges of the process. Here we sum up some of the important advantages of financial planning for retirement.

✓ It provides a clear-cut blueprint of your finances during retirement and enables you to strike the right balance between savings and spending.

✓ It can relatively insulate you from the vagaries of inflation, market volatilities, falling returns, etc.

✓ It empowers you to take good care of yourself and your loved ones.

✓ Optimum planning ensures optimum use of resources, thereby enabling you to bequeath a decent estate to your kith and kin.

✓ It attempts to make your golden years rather dull by taking away financial suspicions, surprises and suspense.

✓ Financial planning process not just makes you financially independent but also makes you aware that you are independent. And that makes the difference.

Accumulation and Expending Stages

Financial planning for retirement can be categorised into accumulation and expending stages. The first stage is the pre-retirement phase when we save for retirement, and the second stage is the post-retirement phase when we require a regular income. The financial planning process for retirement essentially aims to manage the factors influencing accumulation and expending stages. It attempts not merely to counterbalance these two phases but also to create a reasonable surplus for contingencies of the post-retirement phase.

Many people have a propensity to balance accumulation and expending phases theoretically with reference to the prevailing indicators. They are usually more prone to go by the current estimates of many unpredictable factors such as life expectancy, inflation and interest rates. These apparently apt estimates cannot be too reliable to guarantee our financial security in the far-away future. So here, merely balancing savings with the projected expenses may not be an infallible strategy.

To work out a reliable strategy, we can take a cue from this famous saying of Archimedes, *"Give me a long enough lever and I can lift the earth."* What he meant was that if he could stand far enough away from the earth he could use a lever to move the earth. His point was that we could lift anything with a long enough lever by shifting the fulcrum to the right position.

We can apply this simple yet foolproof concept to plan our finances for retirement. Here our lever is our indefinite lifespan and the fulcrum is the retirement age. We simply need to shift the fulcrum to the right to expand the left side of the lever, i.e., the accumulation phase that can provide more than sufficient leverage to take care of the financial concerns of the post-retirement life. The following diagram distinctly depicts the rewards of stretching the known and executable accumulation phase to adequately provide for the relatively unknown and dubious post-retirement phase. Here we are shifting only the retirement age, assuming all other variables like savings amount and interest rate at the same level.

<u>Retirement Reserves – Standard Retirement Age</u>

30   << Age Years >>   90
60

Accumulation   Expending Phase

<u>Retirement Reserves – Extended Retirement Age</u>

30   << Age Years >>   90
70

Accumulation Phase   Expending Phase

In the second case, accumulation phase can potentially boost retirement reserves to more than double as compared to the first case. The concept of time value of money plays a part in providing more than proportionate advantage in the second case. In addition, the duration of expending phase is much less in the second case.

We know that the retirement planning process looks

at many variable factors such as age when you start saving, monthly savings amount, return on investments, retirement age, expenses during retirement, inflation and market dynamics. The planning process is also influenced by many personal factors, like family responsibilities, health concerns, personal goals, preferred lifestyle and the rest. But the two factors, viz. Present age when you start saving for retirement and Retirement age, can really make a big difference to your accumulation endeavours, as you will find hereunder.

Early Saver Advantage

In the process of financial planning for retirement, the most important point to keep in mind is the power of compounding. This can do wonders to your retirement corpus if you have a long way to go before you retire. The benefits of starting early to secure your financial future cannot be overstated. This is the best antidote to meet the challenges of longer life span and dwindling returns on the financial investments. It gives you a good head start owing to the time value of money in conjunction with long duration.

You may be surprised to note that if you start saving at the age of 20 at a return of 20% per annum, you need to save less than $2 per month to retire at the age of seventy with one million dollars. Employed people invariably appreciate the benefits of long-term savings. They exercise thrift and start saving early in career to ensure that retirement does not become a financial nightmare. In fact, they work out retirement needs early in career and save accordingly for the retirement years. The following table quantifies the benefits of starting early to save for your retirement. It shows the amount you need to save every month to accumulate a million dollars by the time of retirement. The first column shows the years you need to save and the second, third, and fourth columns give the amount you need to save every month to amass one million dollars at the interest rate of 5%, 10% or 15% respectively.

Monthly Savings Required to Accumulate One Million

Savings Period	Interest Rate (%) Savings every month ($)		
(Years)	5%	10%	15%
5	15081	13650	12360
10	6625	5229	4104
15	3862	2623	1751
20	2520	1455	813
25	1746	847	392
30	1254	507	192
40	690	188	47
50	398	72	12

Extending Career

The structure of this chapter mandates me to discuss pure money matters influencing retirement finances. Yet unable to restrain myself, I reiterate that the best strategy is to continue to work beyond the traditional retirement age to derive optimum health and financial benefits. This way you can extend the accumulation phase, which not only increases the savings but also shrinks the distribution phase as well as the financial needs during retirement. Even if you have missed on the early saver advantage, this provides you a chance to make up for the lost opportunity. We try to elaborate this with the help of a hypothetical example.

For the sake of simplicity, let us assume that a person aspires to provide for 30 years in retirement after working for 30 years. He plans to provide for his inflation-adjusted retirement expenses from pension and other resources. But he anticipates that his retirement income deficiency will be practically $100,000 per annum, which he wants to balance out with an annuity. With a view to meet this shortfall, he intends to save $1,000 per month @ 8% from age 35 until age 60 when he will retire (column A). But then, his financial planner works out that he needs $1.13 million at the time of retirement to buy an annuity of $100,000 per annum @ 8% for 30 years whereas his savings will accumulate to only $0.88 million. He will face a deficit of $0.25 million at the time of retirement.

Retirement Funds Worksheet

Particulars	Standard Retirement A	Early Saver B	Extended Career C	Early + Extended D
Accumulation Phase:				
Savings Started at Age:-	35	30	35	30
Retirement Age:-	60	60	70	70
Savings Period-years	25	30	35	40
Annual Savings	12000	12000	12000	12000
1. Retirement Funds @ 8% = million $	**0.88**	**1.36**	**2.07**	**3.11**
Distribution Phase:				
Retirement Period- years (up to 90 years)	30	30	20	20
Retirement needs/ Annuity (Amount $ p.a.)	100000	100000	100000	100000
2. Sum Payable for Annuity @ 8% = million $	**1.13**	**1.13**	**0.98**	**0.98**
(1 – 2) Surplus for inheritance = million $	**-0.25**	**0.23**	**1.09**	**2.13**

Let us take the case B wherein he opts to avail early saver advantage and intends to save from age 30 instead of age 35. In this case, his retirement savings will increase to $1.36 million that is sufficient to meet the requirement of $1.13 million at the time of retirement.

Next alternative is the case C wherein he prefers to extend his career by another 10 years after the scheduled retirement date. Here he will save for 35 years and spend 20 years in retirement. In this case, his retirement kitty will swell to $2.07 million as against the requirement of $0.98 million at the time of retirement. He will have a surplus of $1.09 million at the time of retirement, which he can earmark for his loved ones.

Now take the case D in which he intends to take early saver advantage as well as extended career benefits. Here his retirement capital will add up to $3.11 million that is more than three times his retirement needs. Retirement funds worksheet on the previous page clearly illustrates these examples.

As is clear from the above, starting early and extending career can give you an incredible financial advantage to make your golden years truly golden. You should analyse your own accumulation and expending stages by incorporating your estimates in the above table. You can refer online calculators or tables for 'future value of annuity' and 'present value of annuity' to compute retirement corpus and sum payable for annuity respectively. In case of any clarification or for getting your personal worksheet of accumulation and expending stages, you should contact your financial advisor. After appreciating the impact of early saving and extended career on retirement funds, we take up the essential steps involved in the process of fortifying your financial future.

8

Fortifying Your Financial Future

People are living longer than before. Yet, a few are still not preparing themselves to sufficiently provide for extra golden years. Some people are closing the eyes to the changed circumstances by clinging to the outdated notions, which were pertinent when retirement period and financial needs were significantly less.

However, more and more people are realising the need to be financially independent throughout their lives. With financial independence and increase in the disposable income, retirees can opt for an independent life and carve an impressive identity of their own in retirement. Optimal financial planning let them live a life of their own, enjoying their space and sense of dignity. Most people appreciate the importance of retirement planning and often brood over it, albeit in an unstructured manner. Many are now realising the need to establish a definite plan for an honourable subsistence during the later years as they do not expect state and others to bear the burden of their second childhood. Even in the developed countries, the responsibility of financial planning for retirement is shifting away from the state and towards the individual citizen. With an eye to ensure financial security during retirement, we discuss here below five important steps in the process of retirement planning.

Envisioning Retirement

Before you can effectively develop a financial plan for your post-retirement years, you need to figure out what is your definition of golden retirement. Understanding your motivations for the contented post-retirement life will better prepare you to achieve your goals. Then you can wisely proceed to quantify cost implications of your desired lifestyle in retirement.

At this stage, you ought to envision your desired lifestyle in retirement. You have to be well aware of your own definition of a comfortable retired life that will make you and your family happy during your golden years. In essence, you have to create a vision of your perfect retirement and determine what your version of happiness will cost. Next, you need to explore how you can organise your finances in order to pay for that happiness. This will facilitate you to review your financial needs during retirement as well as stimulate your thinking on how to realign your capital along the lines of your retirement vision.

Reviewing Personal Financial Status

Periodically you are supposed to review your personal financial status, as a routine part of your money management regimen. Here it entails revisiting your financial status from the sole perspective of retirement planning to ensure financial security during retirement.

Your retirement vision will enable you to prioritise various components of your personal financial status in proportion to your retirement needs and desires. At various stages in your life, your needs vary thereby prompting you to accord different priorities to the various components of your capital. In the early stages of career, one can afford to be aggressive in investments, which incidentally suits well at that stage to fulfil the long-term retirement objectives. But one has to gradually shift the gears on the way to retirement. One should adopt a neutral approach during middle age that will eventually give way to a more conservative approach in the last stage of work life. The idea is to invest retirement finances in such a way that balance gradually shifts towards fixed return investments over a period of time. This typical pattern has become the hallmark of retirement planning because it creates an optimal balance between wealth creation and retirement objectives.

The following table illustrates a basic assets prioritisation model at various life stages.

Retirement Reserves — Assets Prioritisation Model

Age/Priority → ↓ Assets	30's	40's	50's	60's
House	Medium	High	High	High
Equity	High	High	Medium	Low
Fixed return	Low	Medium	Medium	High
Life insurance	Medium	Medium	High	Medium
Health insurance	Low	Medium	High	High
Annuity	Low	Medium	Medium	High

The above-mentioned general indicators are changeable depending on the various personal factors. These priorities just give a broad idea as to how financial status should move forward while traversing different stages of life cycle.

As it happens, your priorities will be influenced by your unique set of circumstances, such as financial status, family members and their priorities, adequacy of retirement nest egg, your obligations, probable inheritance, need and desire to bequeath, and the rest.

Priorities always differ from person to person, but one factor, i.e., house is on top of the agenda of most people. This shows the commitment of working class towards their retirement vision as the house is invariably the primary factor in the retirement planning process.

Estimating Expenses

In order to prepare adequately for your retirement years, you should know or at least have an inkling of your monthly expenses. You need to estimate your retirement expenses based on your preferred standard of living and other relevant factors in order to find out what your version of happiness will cost. Experts suggest that you will require 70 to 80 percent of your current expenses after retirement to maintain your lifestyle. This may well be deceptively true in the short term. It cannot be taken for granted, as you cannot precisely forecast many variables such as inflation rate, future requirements, family obligations and healthcare expenses.

In spite of all this, it would help you if you quantify your retirement expenses based on the type of lifestyle you plan to have and the timing of your retirement. The process to identify your retirement needs and desires will make you sentient of your preparedness and guide you to organise your accumulation part accordingly. Remember, some animals and careless people do not prepare for their later years, but wise people plan for the future and enjoy their golden years. Here is a table exemplifying the process of estimating monthly expenses.

Forecasting Retirement Expenses

Monthly Expenses	Amount	Likely Change +/- %	% of Total
Living expenses			25-35
Personal debt payments			0-10
Housing expenses			10-25
Health & family care			15-35
Transport expenses			5-10
Recreational expenses			5-15
Miscellaneous expenses			5-15
Total Expenses			

The above analysis will help you determine the probable status of your expenses during the retirement years. This will give you a reasonable idea of your expense replacement ratio that is the percentage of your pre-retirement expenses replaced during retirement.

Retirement professionals recommend a range from 60 to 80% for this ratio for the majority of employed people. Generally, the lower monthly income entails a higher ratio and vice versa. You need to calculate your applicable ratio to forecast your expenses for the future period. In addition, you should set aside an additional amount for miscellaneous expenses that cannot be planned.

Inflation is a fact of life. And it is one of the biggest problems for the retirees. They cannot control it, and they do not know how it will behave in the future. However, they can adopt a cautious and flexible strategy to better insulate their retirement plan against the negative impacts of inflation.

The impact of inflation can lower the purchasing power of your defined income. So it must be rationally accounted for when planning for retirement. You need to calculate your expenses during retirement with realistic inflation in mind. You can use inflation charts to get an inflation-adjusted estimate of your total expenses. And there are also a variety of online inflation calculators to help you project your future expenses and realistically prepare for retirement.

Impact of Inflation on Expenses in Retirement

Year	Total Expenses @ 4% inflation	Total Expenses @ 8% inflation
2020		
2021		
2023		
2024		
...		
....		
2030		
...		
.....		
2050		

While it is usually better to seek professional help with retirement reckonings, remember that your active involvement will always remain indispensable. You need to keep in mind that no one can precisely estimate your future expenses without considering a broad spectrum of your personal issues. Your personal view of retirement lifestyle and the associated expenses along with inflation estimates will have a lot to do with guesstimating your future expenses more accurately.

Estimating Income

Once you have determined your retirement expenses, the next step is to examine your retirement income situation. It is a simple process of ascertaining your cash inflows during retirement in order to examine the sufficiency and sustainability of these during your lifetime. It cautions you in time by recognising the gap between reality and your retirement vision when your future cash inflows are not in sync with your expense projections.

In order to carry out this step logically, it should be organised into three parts:

➢ Quantifying External Sources of Income

➢ Working out Income Deficiency

➢ Examining Personal Sources

Quantifying External Sources of Income

We can broadly classify the sources of retirement income as external and personal. The external sources primarily consist of employers' pension and state benefits. The external sources of income vary significantly from case to case depending on the employers' policies and applicable state benefits, yet they are more or less defined for an individual. Even though these benefits are a function of several factors such as retirement age, status, self-contributions and the like, they can be considered as stable in nature for an individual because these are typically not arbitrary. An individual may not have much control over these since the external authorities govern these, but s/he must fully understand these to take maximum advantage of these benefits. In view of the predetermined character of the external sources of income and adequate awareness of these among beneficiaries, they do not deserve further discussion. Nevertheless, it is important to determine these correctly in order to quantify retirement income deficiency to meet the estimated expenses.

Working Out Income Deficiency

Retirement income deficiency is simply the difference between the defined external sources of income and the estimated expenses during retirement. Most employed people do not experience significant income deficiency because they are innately thrifty with money. They are used to live a simple and responsible life. And they inculcate the same values in their children, who are generally self-supporting at the time of their retirement. More often than not, they fulfil most of their responsibilities by the time they retire. But in a few cases, the income deficiency is likely to be considerable. Whether this is owing to the deficient external sources of income or due to the higher anticipated expenses, they have to bridge the gap on their own from their personal resources. Now we discuss how one should use the personal sources to offset the income deficit.

Examining Personal Sources

There are two common methods to make up the income deficiency from the personal resources– the capital preservation method and the capital utilisation method. Unique circumstances of an individual will determine whether one should go for any one of the methods or an appropriate combination of the two. The need and desire to bequeath assets to the kith and kin favours the preservation method whereas retirement needs may perhaps press for the capital utilisation method. However, one needs to strike a balance between the two considering all the pertinent personal factors.

When you opt for the capital preservation method to meet the shortfall in income, you have to depend on the returns from your investments. This method requires a substantial capital base at the time of retirement. You should make an estimate of the future value of your investments and other assets at the scheduled time of retirement. This will give an indication of sufficiency or otherwise of your retirement corpus to generate adequate income. Here are some common sources of income.

✓ Interest returns on fixed income instruments

✓ Dividends on equity holdings

✓ Rental income from real estate

✓ Trading/Arbitrage income from investments

✓ Income from securities lending

✓ Profit from writing 'out of money' call/put options on self holdings

The capital utilisation method notionally reckons that all the assets will be liquidated to meet the income deficiency during retirement. However, people usually adopt a gradual and staggered approach even if they decide to liquidate all the assets for their retirement needs. Some of the options preferred by people are discussed hereunder.

Cashing Investments: One can make up the shortfall in retirement income by gradually selling investments. One needs to update the personal financial status in order to make a viable and cost efficient plan to liquidate investments. Depending on the personal financial status, i.e., the type and nature of assets, a bankable strategy can be worked out to maximise the cash inflows besides ensuring the continuity of the income. One may consider converting investments including the cash value of life insurance to cash and opt for fixed return instruments or an annuity to ensure steady cash inflows. One has to keep in mind several factors such as age, health situation, net assets, family situation and so on to devise a suitable and lasting strategy.

Annuities: An annuity is a flexible financial instrument that allows accumulating retirement savings and then reaping the benefits of savings in the form of periodic payments or a lump sum payment. Dictionary meaning of annuity is a fixed sum of money paid each year. But, in practice, it refers to periodical payments, generally monthly. It is an excellent tool to ensure lifelong cash inflows to take care of essential needs.

Annuity and pension are similar as both provide regular payments to retired people either by the state or by the employer or from an investment fund. The need for annuity is quite different from that of life insurance. Yet both life insurance and annuity are protective measures. As insurance safeguards a person from the uncertainties of early death, life annuities safeguard a person against the risk of exhausting capital if s/he lives too long. It is an instrument of choice for such people who are not so good at managing their money. Annuities offer much flexibility to retirees who can choose the one that suits their situation from numerous options. There are various types of annuities, e.g. fixed and variable, single life or joint life, refund feature or not, single premium or periodic premium, and so on.

Reverse Mortgage: People who do not have many investments but own a house can opt for reverse mortgage to cope with the retirement income shortfall. We are well conversant with the concept of mortgage or home loan. Reverse mortgage, as the name suggests, in simple words is just the opposite of the mortgage concept. It is aimed to help senior retirees who are *house rich* but *cash poor*. Retirees are not generally eligible for loans, but they can borrow big bucks – either lump sum or as periodic payments against their house.

The borrowers can live in their house as well as receive cash instalments to meet the income deficiency for the rest of their life. The spouse can also avail the benefits as a co-borrower, even after the demise of the borrower. Moreover, the borrower is not required to repay the loan, which is repaid through the sale of the house on the borrower's death. The borrowers usually have the option to prepay the loan with interest at any time during the loan tenure. The borrower's heirs can also repay the loan amount with interest and have the mortgage released.

Other Sources: To augment the retirement income,

one can also explore other options, such as increasing the rate of return within the acceptable risk parameters, extending the retirement age, cutting down the retirement expenses, adapting some lifestyle changes, seeking help from family or friends and so on. If time and other factors permit, one should first consider adding to the savings for the retirement period. Though these are strictly personal choices, one may like to weigh the impact as well as the pros and cons of each supplemental income source on the retirement income shortfall before seriously considering these figures in the retirement reckonings.

Managing the Plan

Investors who are flush with funds can afford to take this exercise flippantly. But all are not so fortunate. In many cases, state and employer benefits are not adequate to meet even the necessities. This problem is further compounded by the inflation, which may diminish the purchasing power of fixed pension and/or annuities as well as the nest egg earmarked for the retirement. Duration of retirement is slowly but surely extending, and as such, people are spending more time in retirement. It is expected to go beyond one-third of our life. All these factors necessitate a planned approach to the retirement issues. To get a clear-cut picture of retirement planning, you can now outline your plan broadly in the following format. Understanding the above steps will help you to complete this exercise in a rational manner.

Financial Specifics of Retirement

Particulars	2020's ⇒	2030's ⇒	2040's ⇒
A. Essence of Retirement Vision			
B. Personal Financial Status: - ... - -			
C. Estimated Expenses: - ... - - -....			

Particulars	2020's ⇒	2030's ⇒	2040's ⇒
D. Income Sources: D.1 External sources- - ... -.... D.2 Personal sources- - ... -....			
E. Retirement Income (D.1-C) Surplus+/Deficit-			

While managing your plan, you need to focus on the two aspects— how your numbers stack up for the first year in retirement and how the numbers are likely to fluctuate going forward. These two aspects will give you the sixth sense to take the timely corrective measures to avert the probable problems in retirement. Managing your retirement plan is not just about ensuring your retirement income needs; it also allows you to make the most of market opportunities.

After setting up your retirement plan aimed at making your golden years truly golden, you need to work assiduously towards achieving your retirement objectives. And you should be very clear about the distinction between *'what you need'* and *'what you want'* to get the most from your planning exercise. Periodically, you should also monitor your financial plan to make sure it is on the right track. But you have to follow a somewhat flexible approach while reviewing or revising your plan in the light of latest developments. Remember, a course correction because of minor issues is not always a good idea. Many a times things fall into place as time passes. So be cautiously optimistic while evaluating your progress.

Success with retirement planning is as simple as knowing how to bridge the gap between means and meaning. In the ultimate analysis of financial independence, what is really important is that you could do what truly matters to you even while covering the last lap of your life's journey.

9

Assessing Your Readiness For Retirement

More often than not, retirement comes with anxieties, uncertainties and insecurities. And planning finances for the retirement needs is just one aspect of dealing with these worries. It is not a complete retirement planning. Retirement planning has a lot to do with graceful acceptance of changing realities and adequately preparing ourselves for these realities. In order to make a winning plan for retirement, it is imperative to have a balanced view of these realities and the ability to take these realities in the right perspective. This will help us to prepare well for the future by rationally assessing our readiness for the post-retirement period.

How can we assess our readiness for the retirement transition? This seemingly simple question is not so simple. In fact, it is the most complex question of this book. For the last two decades, I have been seeking a foolproof formula or a dependable method, which can unambiguously assess our readiness for the retirement. But looking for such a formula or method seems like seeking the Holy Grail in view of myriad known and unknown variables impacting an individual's post-retirement life. But then, not finding a perfect yardstick does not mean that we cannot do anything to improve our later life. Our inability to find a perfect way out does not mean none exists.

Then again, there are many methods available in the market proclaiming to gauge the retirement readiness. Most of these deal with mere financial planning for the retirement. Incidentally, they work well particularly for the affluent people who primarily need a solution to their other non-financial concerns. However, a few attempts to provide an elaborate, but somewhat general assessment in a typically non-subjective mode. Even these usually do not serve the intended purpose in a very personal matter like retirement where the objective is to seek a holistic solution to all the retirement concerns. But they do help, particularly by making a person responsive to the retirement issues.

Why It Is Important to Assess Our Retirement Readiness?

The issue of assessing our retirement readiness is not a new challenge. In fact, it has been bothering people for quite some time. But it is gaining currency nowadays as a consequence of latest breakthroughs in the medical sciences promising better lifespan. When we consider retirement in the traditional sense, i.e., the end of career and withdrawal of the person from the work life and try to seek answers to financial issues only, this deceptive query may not appear so daunting. But we may not possibly get a dependable solution if we take into account other important variables like increased life expectancy, health factors, inflation, return on investments, productive use of time after retirement and so on. Moreover, we cannot expect all the variables to behave as we want. We always want to change the variables to suit our wants, instead of following a mechanism to capitalise on the favourable ones and minimise the impact of adverse ones. For example, while dealing with life expectancy, our objective should not be to live as long as possible, but to empower ourselves to lead a happy, meaningful and frailty-free life. We should strive to add quality years to our life, not just years. In short, we may grow old, but we need not get old.

Retirement planning cannot be a simple and unambiguous exercise considering that we live in a world where financial aspects of retirement are usually overstressed at the expense of health, professional and social aspects. We need to create a balanced framework for retirement that accords due importance to all the relevant elements. Such a model can ensure that important retirement issues are judiciously coordinated so that they can harmoniously build on each other. A prerequisite to the success of such a model is to have a better understanding of what constitutes retirement readiness.

Appreciating Retirement Readiness

Do we really know what makes up the retirement readiness? While traditionally retirement is considered more as a financial event, it also implies major changes in the lifestyle. Retirement readiness is not only about finances – it is about family, friends and freedom too. While the personal definition of retirement varies greatly depending on the unique situation of each person, some basic choices characterised by their individualism, independence and indulgence are common to nearly everyone. Financial independence is equally important for the holistic retirement readiness so as to ensure that lifestyle decisions during retirement are made based on choice, not financial constraints.

People who are used to the 20th century's definition of retirement, holistic retirement planning continues to be an alien concept. They boldly and sometimes blindly enter retirement. They do not adequately recognise that there is much more to retirement than mere financial planning and lounging around. As we have discussed earlier, the whole concept of retirement needs to be redefined to align it with the realities of the 21st century in order to make it a progressive march rather than a march to obscurity.

You need to define and redefine your own concept of retirement to befit your vision of the golden years. Many senior people are retiring old notions of what it means to be retired. They are rethinking retirement to supplement or even supplant the old concept of retirement. They are really reinventing retirement to recharge and revitalise their lives. Many people are pursuing their productive passions that draw on the skills, talents and wisdom they have acquired all through their career. They are listening to the call of their cherished calling to rediscover retirement.

Most people are amenable to the new situation. And they are not averse to managing ego and emotions well in an attempt to confidently stand up to the pulls and pressures of a phlegmatic society. They realise that perhaps retirement is the time to put in practice all the lessons learned in their lives. They know that having a constructive mission can make a big difference in their lives. They are ready for a treat, but not for a retreat. They want to rewire, not retire.

Remember, it is time to become the person you have always dreamed of becoming. Just take control of your life. Cultivate the self-love and confidence needed to become the wonderful person that you have always wanted to be and to live the life you have always wanted to live. Just make plans for retirement bearing in mind this important perspective. This will certainly take care of many indeterminable factors to your advantage.

10

Developing a Holistic Plan For Retirement

Detailed and personalised planning is a prerequisite for a contented life in later years. Developing a holistic plan for retirement may be a challenging task, but it is of utmost importance, as it provides you a blueprint of your future life. It shows you the direction and the viable course of action to make the most of your wisdom phase.

But before you effectively develop a holistic plan for your later years, you have to be very clear about your definition of happy retirement. Understanding your motivating forces will better prepare you to ascend to a new plateau of potentiality to achieve your ambitions in retirement. And you need to make a distinction between *'what you must have'* and *'what you would like to have'* to get the most from your retirement plan. Then you can realistically plan to take care of your desired lifestyle to add both quality and quantity to your life.

Originally, we wanted to illustrate an objective framework to facilitate a rational assessment of retirement readiness. But then, we also appreciate that an individual is in the best position to appraise her or his personal issues influencing retirement decisions. Holistic retirement planning is much larger in scope as it entails planning numerous personal issues. Typically, individual factors are always dynamic, particularly when they relate to age 60 as well as age 70. Personal issues and circumstances can make a big difference to the retirement planning. Because various personal factors gain intensity by the simple fact of their interplay, the co-occurrence of negative factors may present strange challenges. Likewise, the cumulative effect of the personal positive factors can give a head start or even a winning edge. Therefore, we decided against a standard, objective framework because it can be counterproductive in some cases. So, after reviewing pros and cons of an objective process in a highly sensitive and largely personal matter like retirement, we decided to keep it an open-ended exercise to enable the learned readers to assume the responsibility of their golden years. However, the following pointers are aimed at empowering you to make a winning future plan.

Regardless of the fact that there is no foolproof way to

get the right retirement plan, you can follow a very simple strategy to overcome this predicament, i.e., carry on your calling and have flexible plans for future. This way both your career and retirement plan supplement each other, as your retirement nest egg multiplies and your biological ageing slows down. Cumulative impact of such a simple approach will definitely put in the shade any specialised and comprehensive retirement plan.

Therefore, my considered suggestion for you is just go for the basics and adapt a simple do-it-yourself approach. A simple and self-acting process is easy to understand, easy to implement and easy to carry on. And remember following a plan is more important than making a complex plan. Therefore, you should follow your own plan to periodically review your readiness for the retirement. This you can do with reference to the following checklists that prompt you to take care of your weak areas. These modular checklists will help you to design your own strategy to gauge your future readiness.

Financial Planning Questionnaire

→ What personal and financial resources do I have to live comfortably in retirement?

→ How much capital do I need to maintain my desired lifestyle in retirement?

→ Can my retirement reserve accommodate

inflation and market cycles?

→ Can I outlive my retirement kitty? Do I have an alternative strategy for such a situation?

→ Will I have enough funds to take care of my healthcare and other new expenses when I retire?

→ Will I get the amount required every month from assured sources?

→ Is my income from personal sources based on capital preservation method or capital utilisation method or a mix of both?

→ Do I have a well-diversified portfolio to safeguard my capital as well as take benefits of market appreciation?

→ How frequently do I need to re-examine my asset allocation considering inflation and market fluctuations?

→ Have I prepared my income-expense budget and cash flow statements for the retirement?

→ Have I made sufficient provisions to take care of contingencies?

Professional Questionnaire

→ I always had a craving to do something. Can I do that now?

➔ Do I view changeover to retirement as vague and hazy proposition? Or my roadmap is clear and exciting?

➔ How much do I need to work? Am I ready to work that much?

➔ Am I retiring at the right time considering my obligations?

➔ Have I adequately explored the job market or self-employment opportunities?

➔ Have I considered the option of working part-time?

➔ What ought to be a desirable and realistic work schedule for my later years?

➔ Do I have a job search strategy or business plan ready for the golden years?

➔ Have I identified a placement agency or a career-planning organisation catering to my area of expertise?

➔ Do I fully recognise the value of continuing career vis-à-vis consequences of quitting work life?

➔ Does the idea of retirement stimulate me or dishearten me?

➔ Can I retire to enjoy a relaxed and easy

lifestyle, which may include some kind of work?

→ What are the views of my family members and friends on this issue?

Lifestyle Questionnaire

→ Do I feel excited about retirement? ...Why?

→ Do I feel anxious about retirement? ...Why?

→ Do I look at the transition to retirement as a manageable or an ambiguous process?

→ Have I finalised my home? Do I want to relocate to a new area?

→ Do I need to care about relatives and friends in my retirement planning?

→ Are my spouse and other family members ready for my retirement?

→ What can I do just for me after retirement?

→ Have I considered how retirement will influence my health?

→ What is my main health problem and how can I alleviate it?

→ Do I fully appreciate the impact of health and lifestyle issues on life expectancy?

→ Have I understood the important changes I am going to experience after retirement?

→ Can I avert the unpleasant changes, or at least soften their impact?

→ Do I have emotional and psychological resources to live the lifestyle of my choice in retirement?

→ Is my estate planning and will up-to-date considering all probable situations?

→ How will I spend my time in retirement as I have relied on my work place for social contact and psychological fulfilment?

→ Do I have some social activities in mind to keep myself busy after retirement?

→ Who will I be after retirement? Will I like my post-retirement status?

Given that retirement readiness is a very personal situation, you are not supposed to restrict your retirement readiness universe to the above-mentioned checklists. These checklists are intended to stimulate your thinking as you start your retirement planning. They cannot be a substitute for personal retirement planning; individual considerations can make a big difference. So, you need to incorporate your specific concerns in the above checklists to make it a personalised as well as a panoptic exercise. When your retirement plans are specifically customised to your retirement vision, you are on the way to a contented and satisfied retired life. By brainstorming over a virtually simulated exercise, you can aptly appreciate your likely challenges of retirement as well as your preparation for the later years. This is important to psychologically prepare for your future life.

The above-mentioned questions may look like simple questions, yet they require time and focus to find the real answers. This exercise will help you to shortlist your own checklist of weak points where you need to prime yourself to get the most from your golden years.

What we intend to achieve is to get the people take responsibility for their golden years. We want to encourage them to recognise what is holding them back from carrying on or even extending their success march. And when people wisely realise that their main impediments have roots in the misguided notions of retirement, they ignore their unreal barriers and get ready to manage the real barriers. Being adept at solution finding, they know how to deal with their identified real concerns.

While seniors are generally good at taking care of their retirement concerns, they often disregard the importance of time management and updating their knowledge in their second career journey. So while contemplating retirement, you should not entirely depend on your relatives and friends to constructively spend your leisure time. And remember that once you lose touch with your area of expertise, you cannot rely on your expertise and self-confidence for long. So, you need to clearly reflect on how you wish to spend your golden years. With a positive and constructive action plan, you cannot only preserve your knowledge and authority, but can also enhance your status in the society. You can only count on yourself to pursue the right activities and lifestyle to achieve fulfilment and happiness so that you can be a good example to those around you. By continuing your career journey in retirement, you not only take good care of your financial and health aspects, but also enjoy longer and productive life full of meaningful work, activities and happiness.

By brainstorming over the previously mentioned issues and exploring pertinent options, you will be able to take well-informed retirement decisions. Any activity that stimulates you to continue active lifestyle is vital to your retirement planning. The holistic retirement planning is an encouraging and energising tool so long as one remembers it is not an end in itself. Retirement planning is meant to be efficient, not sufficient; and flexible, not fixed.

Remember the saying, "Wisdom is knowing what to do next; virtue is doing it." And no one else can do it for you. So, bestir yourself to prevent anecdotage (anecdote dotage), where all one does is to relate stories about *the good, old days*. Bestir yourself to leverage age. By leveraging your rich experience, you can make it the best period of your life. Take this challenge so that you can gladly face God to say that your life has been well lived.

LIST OF TABLES AND ILLUSTRATIONS

LIST OF TABLES AND ILLUSTRATIONS

www.ingramcontent.com/pod-product-compliance
Lightning Source LLC
Chambersburg PA
CBHW050353280326
41933CB00010BA/1451